(Second Edition)

A Manual on
Cardiac Resuscitation

By

ROBERT M. HOSLER, M.D., F.A.C.S.
Cleveland, Ohio

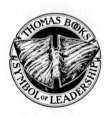

CHARLES C THOMAS · PUBLISHER
Springfield · Illinois · U.S.A.

CHARLES C THOMAS • PUBLISHER
BANNERSTONE HOUSE
301-327 East Lawrence Avenue,
Springfield, Illinois, U.S.A.

*Published simultaneously in the British Commonwealth
of Nations by*

BLACKWELL SCIENTIFIC PUBLICATIONS, LTD., OXFORD, ENGLAND

Published simultaneously in Canada by
THE RYERSON PRESS, TORONTO

Library of Congress Catalog Card Number: 57-13258

*Printed in Cape Girardeau, Mo.,
in the United States of America*

DEDICATED
To my wife
Helen Johnson Hosler

FOREWORD

WITHIN THE memory of those of us who have practiced medicine during the last four decades, the mystery of chest surgery has been resolved. The diagnosis of brain lesions and their surgical relief, presently offer as much hope as we formerly associated with pelvic and abdominal surgery. Now, like lightening across the starless heavens of a stormy night, open chest cardiac resuscitation, illuminates the utter hopelessness which has always followed upon the announcement "the heart has ceased to beat, the patient is dead."

The blinding impact of this reality is naturally followed by the recoil, this has never been, this is not realistic. Our professional understanding requires a period of readjustment to the glare. Reason and logic demand the support of clinical demonstration, observed personally, supported by post-operative confirmation before we assent. Because of the nature of the issue, however, acceptance is quickly replaced by enthusiastic support.

Dr. Claude S. Beck's pioneering efforts in this vital and dramatic field have become an important

part of the History of Medicine. Dr. Robert M. Hosler, his Associate, has presented the logical approach
to the problem, once each month, for almost a decade.
He repeatedly confirms by clinical demonstrations
and post-operative reports the inescapable conclusion that "the hope" of open chest cardiac resuscitation has become a blazing reality.

For those who would question these statements
as over-enthusiastic we would suggest: Experience
the feel of a dog's beating heart within your hand.
Cause this heart to fibrillate and see the blood pressure drop to zero. Note the restoration of this pressure to normal in the electromanometer, activated
solely through the purposeful, repeated pressure of
your fingers and thumb. See the procedure repeated
twenty times by twenty different hands upon the
same heart. Observe the automatic beat at the end
of this sequence. Then place the question—"Can I
ever again, deny a heart, which has ceased to beat,
this one and only chance of survival?"

Your answer will confirm the fact that you are
now oriented in the glare of this new, this single
hope, of one who is functionally dead. "May he rest
in Peace" through the Grace of God, may now become—"Arise and walk."

PALUEL J. FLAGG. M.D.
September 22, 1957

FOREWORD

THE DEVELOPMENT of the resuscitation technique outlined in this manual is one of the best pieces of research and development I have ever witnessed. Although it is so simple in its present form that it can be learned in a few hours, its development took many hundreds of hours in the laboratory and a great deal of learning things that "were not so."

It is impossible to put a value on this work for one cannot estimate how much a human life is worth. If all surgeons learn the technique outlined in this manual, there can be no question the savings to society will be of major importance. The immense effort and careful, ingenious work of Doctor Robert M. Hosler and Doctor Claude S. Beck will be paid off in lives otherwise lost.

JAMES H. RAND, III, Sc.D. (Hon.)
Trustee Cleveland Area Heart Society

September 1, 1952

ix

PREFACE TO THE SECOND EDITION

R ESUSCITATION which dates back to antiquity has shown considerable development in the past few years. At the time of the publication of the first edition it was discreetly felt that these life-saving principles should apply only to those persons who die in or near the operating room. However, it was stated that "Future developments will make it practical to enlarge the scope of this life-saving procedure."

The time has now come to expand its frontier and to consider its successful application in many situations. Resuscitation is in its infancy, and it will continue to expand in its practical application.

The widespread circulation of this small book is a source of inspiration and gratification to the author. Slowly the domain of cardiac resuscitation is no longer associated with cardiac surgery, but rightfully has become a useful tool of all surgeons as well as the medical and dental professions in general. The question now arises whether or not it will become an adjunct to those non-professional groups who are technically trained in resuscitation, those most likely to reach the victim first.

The author wishes to thank Doctor Robert A. Hingson for the ingenious and enthusiastic chapter, Oxygen, the Fuel of Life, which deals with respiratory resuscitation.

I am indebted to Miss Verna Metzger for typing the manuscript. My thanks are extended to Miss Rose Beckman for aid with the bibliography. I am greatly appreciative of the conscientious proof reading which was done by my wife.

R. M. H.
June 30, 1957.

PREFACE

IT IS THE PURPOSE of this handbook to present a practical method for combating one of the most terrifying emergencies which can ever confront the surgeon and anesthetist in the operating room. Practicing physicians are interested in practical methods, and any attempt to delve too deeply into theory in this problem may lead to confusion. A crystal clear understanding of the problem and a step by step application of the procedure will often result in saving a human life. At times it is a downright simple task —in fact so simple on certain occasions that it leads one to speculate that many have succumbed who might have been saved.

This subject has begged for recognition for at least fifty years and it is difficult to understand why this vital matter was not taught or mentioned in most of the medical schools.

It is presumed that there is a definite need for a handbook upon this subject, as the author has had numerous requests for some type of manual which will give a concise overall portrayal of the treatment and understanding a cardiac arrest. These requests have been for a reference book which may serve as a "refresher" and have come chiefly from those doctors and anesthetists who already have taken the course in Cardiac Resuscitation which has been presented in Cleveland, Ohio, since November, 1950.

This book is not necessarily intended for the accomplished thoracic surgeon, but it will fulfill the needs of doctors carrying out all types of surgery. The concept that any doctor is and should be capable of carrying out this resuscitative procedure is developed. It emphatically specifies the correct things to do almost as in a recipe or a chemical formula. The repetition of important basic facts has been found necessary in the teaching of this life-and-death matter. Although the circumstances may not always be ideal, any reasonable attempt at cardiac resuscitation is invariably justified.

The author wishes to thank the following friends for their help: Mr. Lewis Zender of the U. S. Steel Corporation; Mr. V. O. McCreight of University School; Mrs. John B. Dempsey; and Doctor Frederick A. Coller, whose confidence in this work was highly encouraging. The support given by the following colleagues in our Course in Cardiac Resuscitation is greatly appreciated: Doctors Fred R. Mautz, Donald Hale, B. B. Sankey, Robert Hingson, David Leighninger, James Rand, and Kenneth Wolfe.

My mentor, teacher, and esteemed friend, Claude S. Beck, has done more than any other single in-

dividual in bringing to the profession practical principles of resuscitation.

The late Doctor R. J. Whitacre kindly consent-
ed to write the chapter on Danger Signals heralding
this catastrophe. The author is extremely grateful
for this, as an experienced anesthesiologist is the
only person qualified to present this phase.

The bibliography is not extensive on this subject; nevertheless, the author has tried to be fairly
complete in it, and if any name has been omitted, it
is an oversight and has not been intentional. No
formal system of references has been used; consequently, the bibliography is found at the end of the
chapters and at the end of the manual.

R. M. H.

December 1, 1952

CONTENTS

FOREWARD vii

PREFACE TO SECOND EDITION xi

PREFACE xiii

    I. INTRODUCTION 3

    II. HISTORY 7

    III. GENERAL CONSIDERATIONS 16

    IV. ADDITIONAL CONSIDERATIONS 21

    V. INCIDENCE 26

    VI. MECHANISM OF THE HEART BEAT 33
        Development of Cardiac Standstill ... 36
        Ventricular Fibrillation 39

    VII. OXYGEN AND THE BRAIN 44

    VIII. ETIOLOGY 52
        Predisposing Factors Contributing to
          Cardiac Arrest Prior to the Operation . 54
        Drugs 54

Cardiac Disease 58

Vital Capacity 58

Position of the Patient 59

Cardiac Filling 60

Anemia 61

Nutrition 62

Anxiety 62

Shock 63

Speed of Induction 63

Errors 63

Temperature 64

Racial Predisposition 64

Other Predisposing Factors Possibly Present During the Operation 65

Duration of Operation 65

Hypoxia 66

Reflex Stimulation 66

Manipulation of the Heart 67

Anesthetic Agents 68

Tracheal Obstruction 71

Carbon Dioxide 71

Miscellaneous Factors 72

IX. PREVENTIVE MEASURES 74

Intratracheal Intubation 84

X. DANGER SIGNALS OF CARDIAC ARREST 88

CONTENTS   xix

XI. EQUIPMENT FOR RESUCITATION 94
    Equipment for Anesthetist 94
    Resuscitation Kit 94
    Necessary Drugs 96
    Defibrillator 96
    Mechanical Respirator 103
    Equipment 106

XII. STEPS IN CARDIAC RESUSCITATION 107

    Things Not to Do 111
    Re-establishment of the Oxygen System
        (the Emergency Act) 112
    Restoration of the Heart Beat 119
    Cardiac Standstill 119
    Ventricular Fibrillation 121
    Step by Step Program of Action for Re-
        establishment of the Oxygen System 129
    Step by Step Program for Restoration of
        Heart Beat 130

XIII. METHODS OF CARDIAC MASSAGE 131
    Massage with Intact Pericardium 132
    Subdiaphragmatic Approach 132
    Transdiaphragmatic Approach 134
    Transthoracic Approach 134
    Massage with One Hand 134
    Massage with Both Hands 136

Assisted Massage 139
Rate of Massage 139
Suction Cup Massage 140

XIV. CLOSURE OF THE CHEST 141

XV. POST-OPERATIVE MANAGEMENT 145

XVI. RESULTS 152

XVII. FIELDS OF APPLICATION 154
Acute Coronary Insufficiency with Mec-
hanism Death 156
Electrocution 158
Drowning 160
Heart Block 162
Asphyxia 163
Paralysis of Respiratory Center 164
Air Embolism 164
Acute Carbon Monoxide Poisoning 165
New Born Infants 167

XVIII. THE COURSE IN CARDIAC RESUSCITATION ... 168

XIX. OXYGEN, THE FUEL OF LIFE 180
Fundamental Considerations 185
Differences in Children and Adults 193

XX. LEGAL ASPECTS 195

BIBLIOGRAPHY 199

INDEX 203

A MANUAL ON
CARDIAC RESUSCITATION

I

INTRODUCTION

by

Claude S. Beck, M.D.

Knowledge of resuscitation methods should be considered as a requirement for every surgeon and every anesthetist. All specialty boards in surgery, the American College of Surgeons, and all training centers in surgery should make this knowledge a requirement. Methods for resuscitation are in existence. The fundamentals of the procedure are clear and simple. Application of these methods to patients who die in the operating room is a demand that society is entitled to make of the operating surgeon, the anesthetist and the institution where the surgery is done. *Success* in the application of resuscitation methods cannot be considered as a requirement of the surgeon, anesthetist and institution. However, *an attempt* to carry out resuscitation, whether it be *successful* or *unsuccessful* can be considered as a reasonable requirement of these three agencies.

These statements represent my own personal

opinions. For our time, the middle of the twentieth century, most surgeons and anesthetists and almost all institutions would refuse to accept these statements as requirements. Perhaps the time is not ripe for this acceptance of responsibility. The movement towards acceptance of responsibility has been slow. In 1921, one of the famous hospitals of this country called in the fire company to help out in one of these crises (for a pulmotor). The hospital staff were not able to carry on. Few hospital superintendents are aware that they have responsibility to provide the necessary apparatus for resuscitation. Few chiefs of surgery feel obligated to give demonstration courses on resuscitation using the dog for demonstration. Few hospitals put on a drill (like a fire drill) so that the personnel will know what to do when the crisis occurs.

Is there any justification to say that it is a crime to let any patient with a good heart and a good pair of lungs die in the operating room without any attempt at resuscitation? Is it inertia and lack of understanding by those in surgery and in hospital administration? The methods exist. Resuscitation can be successful if done right.

Several years ago the Cleveland Area Heart Society established a course in resuscitation for surgeons and anesthetists under my direction. The purpose of the course was to make resuscitation into a practical step-by-step procedure. Before the course was started the elementary components of the resuscitation procedure were clear. Innumerable repetitions of the procedure have given these elementary components the authenticity of history. These components are facts and history gives them substance. The components are (1) restoration of the oxygen system; and (2) restoration of the heart beat. The restoration of the oxygen system consists of getting oxygen into the lungs and then circulating it to the brain. This is the emergency act. After it has been started and kept in operation the restoration of the heart beat can be carried out without special reference to time. Parts 1 and 2 are separate and distinct steps. They must not be confused. The techniques used in Part 2 must not displace the technique of Part 1, and after Part 1 has been instituted it must be kept in operation until Part 2 has been successfully accomplished.

This separation makes it possible to assign proper importance to the various acts that might be taken in the resuscitation procedure. For example, no one would give an intra-arterial transfusion or take time for an electrocardiogram or inject adrenalin into the heart and then wait for a response when Part 1 should be gotten under way. This separation of the procedure makes such acts obviously wrong, and it can be readily understood why they are wrong. In my opinion this separation of the procedure into these two parts is an important contribution to successful application to patients.

This treatise by Dr. Hosler will fill an important need in surgery. It follows the broad outline of our course. It presents information that should be known before and not after the crisis occurs. The time should be past when we surgeons turn these emergencies over to someone else to take care of (like the fire company) . We should take care of them ourselves.

II

HISTORY

THE TERM "cardiac arrest" is a relatively new technical expression; however, the condition it describes and its connotations are intimately associated with anesthesia. With the successful introduction of ether and chloroform anesthesia in 1846 and 1847, respectively, there soon occurred poorly understood incidents of collapse under anesthesia. It appears that the second and third patients to whom chloroform anesthesia was administered died of what today would be called cardiac arrest.

The first anesthetic[1] death was recorded on January 28, 1848. It soon became apparent to the pioneers in anesthesia that great care had to be exercised in the administration of these useful stupefying and pain relieving gases, if their inherent benefits were to be realized. We are familiar with the fact that Queen Victoria was given chloroform anesthesia during its early development. It is interesting to reflect that if tragedy on this historic occasion had resulted, would it have impeded the progress of anesthesia twenty-five years or more?

From time immemorial man has succumbed to

some form of asphyxia. It is reasonable to assume that down through the ages before written history there have been attempts and occasional successful revivals. In this twentieth century the resuscitation problem still exists.

It may be assumed that asphyxial episodes have been common to man since earliest times. He has been subject to suffocation by mechanical strangulation, foreign bodies in the throat, drowning and by smoke (if not actually subject to carbon monoxide asphyxia). These experiences are reflected in the myths, legends and folk-tales of the world; and since such tales are believed to be the product of human experience, it may be concluded that even aside from medical records, there is abundant evidence of asphyxia as a cause of death. From common cause of death; strangulation, drowning, suffocation by smoke, mine gases, fumes from charcoal stoves, fermenting substances, etc. Babes have been asphyxiated at birth or subsequently smothered, accidentally or otherwise, in their bedclothes or wrappings. In the past century and a half, the noxious gases of coal mines, the exhaust fumes of gasoline engines, as well as illuminating gas have replaced the charcoal burner as sources of carbon monoxide. The dangers from ascension to high altitudes in balloons have likewise been replaced by even more serious dangers of stratospheric aviating. General anesthesia likewise carries with it the threat of anoxia.— (From C. B. Courville, *Cerebral Anoxia*)

Schiff,[2] a physiologist, in 1874 was one of the first to record experiments in which he carried out successful heart massage on anesthetized animals whose hearts had been quiescent up to 11½ minutes. At this time not all resuscitation endeavors were confined to the laboratory. In 1889 Niehaus of Berne was the first to attempt resuscitation of the human heart by manual massage. Maag[2] in 1900 had the first partial success with a human subject. His patient survived 11 hours after the restoration of the heart beat. Starling[3] and Lane reported the first successful instance of a human case of cardiac resuscitation in 1902. Lane performed an abdominal operation on a 65-year-old man. The heart unexpectedly stopped. Artificial respiration was instituted; Lane massaged the heart via the sub-diaphragmatic approach and soon a satisfactory pulse was obtained. Normal respirations did not return for twelve minutes. Inglesburd[2] reported in 1903 that two years previously he had successfully resuscitated a human patient in the operating room. In England the name of Hamilton Bailey is outstanding because of his contributions to this field.

In this country, a considerable amount of experimental and clinical investigation was done in Cleveland, Ohio. The pharmacologist, Sollman, became interested in resuscitation. He stated that one of the best stimulants to an arrested heart in the laboratory was adequate filling of the heart and stretching of the muscle fibers and coronary vessels. Crile[5] and Dolley published their laboratory work on the resuscitation of dogs in 1906. It is interesting that two of their conclusions are so notable today: (1) "the dogs could be uniformly resuscitated without evidence of brain injury up to five minutes after cessation of the heart beat"; (2) "the probable success of resuscitation is greater in an inverse relation to the lapse of time after death."

Crile[6] in 1904 reported the successful resuscitation of a 12-year-old girl following the perfusion of adrenalin solution into the brachial artery. He dramatically refers to this in his biography as "Death and Resurrection." He held the perfusion bottle high above his head and much to his surprise there was a violent shaking of the chest and bright red blood began spurting into the bottle with each heart beat. The operation for removal of a cerebellar tumor was then continued. He personally followed this girl's career for many years.

In 1926, while doing a gallbladder operation, Jackson* of Cleveland succeeded in bringing back to life by cardiac massage a prominent manufacturer who was the father of ten children. This man lived a normal life for eighteen years thereafter.

By clinical and laboratory observation it became apparent that successful restoration of the heart beat could be accomplished when the heart was found in a quiescent state or at a standstill. Many times it was found in a quivering or fibrillating state, and little or nothing could be done to induce the organ to return to a co-ordinated beat. This fact seems to be the stumbling block which retarded the progress in this field. However, two French investigators, Batelli[7] and Prevost, in 1899, successfully

---

*Personal conversation with T. S. Jackson.

brought cats' hearts out of ventricular fibrillation by
the application of 240 volts of alternating electrical
currents. Their work attracted little attention. Today it is accepted that this is relatively easy in the cat
heart. The cat heart will tolerate more injury than
the heart of the dog or human. Is this the reason for
the saying that a cat has nine lives? In this respect,
the heart of the human, the aristocrat of the animals,
lies somewhere between the cat and the dog.

Some twenty-five to thirty years later, Hooker,[8]
Kouwenhoven, Langworthy, and Wiggers reported similar achievements from their laboratories
while experimenting with the dog's heart. Other laboratory investigators had been successful in defibrillation by using the proper combination of the ions,
calcium and potassium. This has had very little practical application in the operating room at the time
of an emergency.

My first introduction to cardiac arrest occurred
while working in the laboratory of Claude Beck on
the experimental problem of cardiac adhesions. The
text books at that time unequivocally stated that
cardiac adhesions were detrimental to the action of
the heart and were often the cause of cardiac hyper-
trophy. The conclusions[10] drawn from these experimental animal studies and autopsy material dis-
proved this theory and were as follows: Cardio-peri-
cardial adhesions per se do not cause cardiac hyper-
trophy. They are not detrimental to the circulatory

system unless they cause constriction, angulation, or torsion of the heart. (The heart may be manipulated parallel to its long axis without undue circulatory embarrassment.)

Part of my time in the laboratory in 1933 was occupied by assisting Beck when he embarked upon what has proved to be his greatest work, that of creating a new blood[11] supply, and redistribution of the blood supply to the heart, to combat nature's foremost killer, namely coronary occlusion. By sheer tenacity, imagination, hard work, and faith he has reached his goal. The hundreds of animal experiments have culminated into a surgical procedure known as the Beck operation. This operation is now being successfully carried out on patients who have coronary insufficiency.

In these early experiments a Goldblatt clamp was applied to one or two of the main coronary trunks, and about every three weeks the small screw head had to be taken down the prescribed number of turns. Rather frequently, and in spite of the fact that heparin was given intravenously at this early date, the dog's heart would go into ventricular fibrillation. Attempts at resuscitation were fruitless. Weeks and months of labor were for naught. Thus resuscitation was introduced into the coronary research problem. Twenty-two years later it was introduced into the clinical coronary problem. (Case viii).

Coincident with this, Beck had the misfortune

of having a patient whose heart went into ventricular fibrillation while he was "peeling" a thickened scar from the surface of her heart to relieve chronic cardiac compression (Pick's disease). Beck became engrossed in the subject of resuscitation and decided to do something about it if only to salvage some of the weeks of labor spent on the laboratory animals. Using published knowledge and developing his own technique, instruments, and principles, he soon was able to salvage or save about fifty per cent of the animals in which ventricular fibrillation had taken place. The results were definitely improved when Beck and Mautz introduced procaine into the procedure to reduce the surface irritability of the heart to external stimuli, and by intravenous administration to decrease the hyperirritability of the heart. Unbeknown to them, Francois-Franck in 1893 referred to the surface application of cocaine to reduce the heart's irritability and to avoid reflexes. In 1904 this same physiologist had studied the value of cocaine to increase the resistance of the heart against ventricular fibrillation caused by electrical currents.

The first successful case of defibrillation of the human heart by electrical shock was carried out by Beck in 1947.[12] The patient was a 14-year-old boy upon whom a three-hour chest operation had just been completed and the skin incision was practically closed. The pulse stopped suddenly and there was no blood pressure. The patient was temporarily dead.

The chest was re-opened and cardiac massage was immediately initiated and carried out for seventy-five minutes. The electrocardiogram at the end of thirty-five minutes was characteristic of ventricular fibrillation. After several series of shocks had been given, procaine was injected into the heart. Following the next shock, feeble coordinated beats were seen. Three hours after defibrillation the patient responded to questioning. This boy has led a normal life since his convalescence.

A practical suction cup electrode defibrillating[13] machine was developed by Beck and Rand after considerable experimentation in 1949.

In 1950 Beck, Rand and Hosler,[14] with the sponsorship of the Cleveland Area Heart Society, inaugurated what is thought to be the first course of its kind and the first concerted attempt by the medical profession to establish a practical educational program for the prevention and treatment of cardiac arrest occurring in the operating room. This course is described in a later chapter.

Why this queer lack of knowledge prevailed in medical educational circles is difficult to explain. This subject from 1902 to 1950 seemed to be in an underground tunnel and then it suddenly emerged into the light of practicality.

BIBLIOGRAPHY

1.   Lahey, F.; Ruzicka, E. R.: *Surg., Gynec. & Obstet.,*

90:108, 1950.
2. Barber, R. F.; Madden, J. L.: *Am. J. Surg., 70*:135, 1945.
3. Starling, E. H.; Lane, W. A.: *Lancet, 2*:1397, 1902.
4. Bailey, H.: Impending Death Under Anes. *Brit. M. J., 2*:84, 1941.
5. Crile, G.; Dolley, D. H.: *J. Exper. Med., 8*:713, 1906.
6. Crile, G.: An autobiography. Vol. I, page 155.
7. Batelli; Prevost: See original bibliography.
8. Hooker, D. R.; Kowenhoven, W. B.; Langworthy, O. E.: *Am. J. Physiol., 103*:444, 1933.
9. Wiggers, C. J.: Circulation in Health and Disease. Fifth Edition.
10. Hosler, R. M.; Williams, J. E.: *J. Thoracic Surg., 5*:629, 1936.
11. Hahn, R. S.; Kim, M.; Beck, C. S.: Revascularization of the Heart. *Am. Heart J., 44*:472, 1952.
12. Beck, C. S., *et al.*: Ventricular Fibrillation of Long Duration Abolished by Electrical Shock, *J.A.M.A., 135*:985, 1947.
13. Beck, C. S.; Rand, J. H.: *J.A.M.A., 141*:1230, 1949.
14. Hosler, R. M.: Training in Cardiac Resuscitation. *Ohio State M. J., 48*:228, 1952.

III

GENERAL CONSIDERATIONS

C ARDIAC ARREST or stoppage of the heart in the operating room is the enigma and challenge of present day surgery and anesthesia. We cannot bury our heads in the sand and ignore this challenge. Every surgeon may at some time be called upon to face the impending death of the patient under anesthesia.

Cardiac arrest can occur under a number of circumstances. It can take place under local or regional anesthesia as well as under general anesthesia. It can happen to the experienced operator who is in the habit of making complicated procedures seem simple, as well as to the beginning intern. Furthermore, it may strike during a simple procedure as well as during a long, complicated one. Cardiac arrest appears almost as frequently to the young as to the old, and as often to a patient with a good heart as to the individual with a known heart impairment.

Its threat haunts all hospitals.

When this terrifying and unexpected incident occurs in a person with a normal heart and a good pair of lungs, it can be likened to turning off the ignition key in an expensive automobile. The car, theoretically, is as good as ever, but unless its motor can be made to function, it is as worthless as a pile of scrap. Such is the case with our patient, who will remain dead unless we can supply the needed "spark."

The primary *problem* in these instances is to keep the brain alive. Unless it is stated often and can be incorporated in one simple sentence, one is likely to lose sight of this BASIC CONSIDERA-TION. The brain can be kept viable* indefinitely by having a small but continuous amount of oxy-genated blood course steadily through its arteries.

A clearer understanding of the length of time of cardiac stoppage is pertinent. There is confusion in reading and making reports on this fundamental consideration. Barber and Madden, among others, have suggested that cardiac arrest is the length of time between the cessation of the heart beat and the re-establishment of the circulation. This does not mean until the heart beat has been restored (this may take hours), but refers to the length of time elapsed until the surgeon gets his hand upon the heart and carries out purposeful manual massage.

It is the intention of this handbook to present positive, essential, and practical methods of dealing with this extraordinary catastrophe. Unless a lucid, clear understanding of the procedure is mastered, the surgeon, when suddenly called upon, may not be

---

*Hill, L.: Reference

equal to the test. A step-by-step plan must be so firmly impressed in his mind, that at any given moment
the correct procedure can be called into use almost
reflexly. ACTION MUST BE IMMEDIATE. One
cannot lean upon consultation in this crisis.

The surgeon cannot take time to think out this
problem. It takes time to cogitate, and during such
a time of stress there is always the chance of error in
human judgment. One must be absolutely right, as
there is only one opportunity for success. In this
league one is not allowed three strikes. The surgeon can be certain of performing the correct procedure only if through previous understanding—or
shall it be called indoctrination?—the action is reduced to a reflex maneuver. The properly developed
reflex will result in action without error.

With a full comprehension of the problem and
the proper application of proven principles, the procedure is relatively simple.

In general, and as of today, these resuscitative
principles apply only to those persons who die in
or near the operating room. Future developments
will make it practical to enlarge the scope of this
life-saving procedure. Research in this subject is not
completed, but with correct institutional planning,
various hospital divisions can be set up to take care
of this crisis when it occurs. (First Ed., 1954.)

Obviously, the best treatment for this condition
is prevention. Every effort that is humanly possible

should be spent in its prevention.* The return to emphasis upon the prevention of cardiac arrest is today like a breath of fresh air. Overemphasis on cardiac resuscitation, if prevention were neglected, could be likened to locking the barn after the horse had been stolen. There is still a job to be done in this field. However, if a surgeon is confronted with this extraordinary situation and hopes to be successful, he must have a definite preconceived plan of action indelibly stamped into his brain. He does not have time to improvise during those precious moments when life hangs in the balance. The time limitation of Three to Five Minutes must be met and overcome if complete recovery is to be obtained.

Not all patients who suffer cardiorespiratory failure in the operating room can be resuscitated. For success, the proper procedure must be executed, and the patient should have a good heart, good lungs, and an adequate blood volume. If any of these are abnormal, resuscitation may not be possible. Patients differ. Some have strong hearts that do not stop easily; others have an unexplainable tendency to fail. The respiratory center shows a variable reaction in different individuals. Some stop breathing more readily than others. The inherited patterns to utilize oxygen efficiently differ.

---

*Paluel Flagg's efforts are outstanding in this field of hypoxia and asphyxia.

Regardless of the situation or condition, it is possible for the physician to take control of the oxygen system for the patient and manage it for several hours, during which time the patient cannot die. After a period of time, the control of the oxygen system must be given back to the patient. If conditions are such that the patient can properly control the system, then the resuscitation will be successful; otherwise he will expire.

In the face of cardiovascular or pulmonary disease, any attempt of resuscitation may seem futile. However, this previously known fact should not deter the surgeon from making a persistent attempt at resuscitation. A pessimistic attitude is to be deplored.* This can no longer be labelled irrational hope.

BIBLIOGRAPHY

1. Hill, L.; Albutt System of Medicine, Vol. 8, p. 262, 1899.

---

*See Case History No. VII and No. VIII.

IV

ADDITIONAL CONSIDERATIONS

CARDIAC RESUSCITATION is still in its infancy. Only within the past six or seven years has it become an acceptable procedure in the operating room.

Death is defined as the cessation of all vital functions without capability of resuscitation. General surgery is now in the fortunate position of being able to challenge and evaluate the word capability, having now in its grasp the ability to restore all the vital functions in countless patients. Whereas formerly cardiac arrest was of itself capable of bringing about such a complete cessation, now that condition can be reversed.

Our conception of so-called death must necessarily undergo new consideration, for the death factor may at times be small and reversible. Like a clock or engine, an arrested heart can be re-activated and it will continue to function for an indefinite period. The precipitating factor at times amounts to a minor mechanical breakdown, the magnitude of which in certain circumstances becomes sufficient to cause cessation of the heart with resulting deterioration of the cerebral cortex and loss of life. This is the decisive and basic problem in resuscitation, namely to keep the brain viable. As the body undergoes deterioration or death, all the organs of the body are not simultaneously rendered incapable of resuscitation. Thus to apply the definition, the body undergoes death not as an unit, but as an orderly progression which is dependent upon the amount of anerobic tissue oxidation which can take place in each organ.

The upper centers of the brain, those phylogenetically developed last, are the most vulnerable to lack of oxygen. Under ordinary conditions these centers will withstand anoxia for three to four minutes before irreversible damage has taken place. The adrenal glands are next in vulnerability to anoxia, followed by the kidneys or liver, then the lower centers of the brain. The heart as a muscular organ is well down this designated ladder of descendency of selective vulnerability. Although it will remain viable it must have oxygenated blood in its coronary system in order to function.

Experience leads us to believe that the time has arrived when resuscitative procedures can and must be included in the treatment of cardiac stoppage[1,2,3] from acute coronary insufficiency. There are now several reports on record of people who have been successfully revived even after suffering apparent death from acute coronary occlusion. Many of these hearts will beat again if given the second chance. Death can occur from minimal myocardial damage.

No doubt there are many similar persons who, if their hearts were given another chance, might function well for a considerable time in the future.* They have good heart muscle except for a tiny area of slight damage. Yater[4] found in his autopsy series of 950 men who died of coronary artery disease in the Armed Forces, that one-third showed no evidence of myocardial damage. Mechanism death occurred in well over 90 per cent of all the victims. These hearts stopped[5] as a result of a difference in electrical potentials resulting from oxygen differentials between the anoxic segment of myocardium and the normally oxygenated myocardium. Electrical currents are produced by differences in oxygen content and its influence upon the cellular electrolytes in adjacent areas of muscle. This might be compared to a small battery, and its potential may overcome the normal electrical impulse originating in the A-V node. If this particular heart has a low threshold of ventricular fibrillation, it can produce a fatality by electrocution, which has been called mechanism death.

When the lumen of a branch of the coronary system is obstructed or significantly reduced in caliber, a state of electrical instability occurs which can be recorded. Hypothetically, there may be a total reduction of blood flow through the heart of five per

---

*Case history VIII.

cent. In other instances there may be a *UNIFORM* reduction of blood flow throughout the coronary system of fifty per cent, yet this heart can be uniformly cyanosed, but it will remain electrically stable and continue to function indefinitely. As paradoxical as it may seem, the difference between life and death in coronary insufficiently can be a small amount of blood. Usually it is a problem of unequal distribution in the myocardium rather than in the amount available. A more even distribution of coronary system flow would prevent or reduce the formation of these marginal areas of dangerous electrical instability. This is the basis for the treatment of coronary insufficiency with the Beck operation.

Resuscitation may under satisfactory circumstances be effectually applied to victims of electrocution, asphyxia, drowning, massive hemorrhage, drugs, (particularly those which have an over-whelming paralyzing effect upon the respiratory center) and air embolism. Resuscitative measures are applicable in the hospital for treating certain new-born infants and in the victims of acute bulbar poliomyelitis who suffer cardiac arrest from anoxia. This tragedy also confronts those who administer drugs of any kind by injection in the home, office or hospital. Time and experience will record the feasibility of resuscitation in well-organized dental offices and possibly in electrical power stations.

BIBLIOGRAPHY

1. Celio, A.: Cardiac Arrest Associated with Coronary Occlusion; Successful Resuscitation. *J. Internat. Coll. Surg., 25:*299, 1956.
2. Mozen, H., *et al.*: Successful Defibrillation of Heart. *J.A.M.A. 162:*11, 1956.
3. Beck, C. S., *et al.*: Fatal Heart Attack and Successful Defibrillation. *J.A.M.A., 161:*434, 1956.
4. Yater, W., *et al.*: A Study of 950 Autopsied Cases From the Armed Forces. *Ann. Int. Med., 34:*352 1951.
5. Brofman, B., *et al.*: Electrical Instability of Heart. *Circulation, 13:*161, 1956.

V

INCIDENCE

Cardiac arrest on the operating table occurs several times each year in every large hospital. Reliable figures on its incidence are not available, as too often in the past these catastrophes were forgotten as soon as possible and the records were not studied or analyzed. Labelled as heart failure, heart attack, or persistent thymus, many of the case records were buried in the archives of the hospitals.

In one town of 60,000 population, an 190-bed general hospital, with its well-trained anesthesia personnel, had eighteen such operating room deaths in seventeen months. One surgeon had six of these cases, and he has stated that the mental anguish and discouragement have been almost enough to persuade him to give up the practice of surgery.

A common estimate is that sudden cardiac stoppage will occur on the average of five times each year in a 700-bed active hospital. Journals relating to anesthesia indicate that it will happen once in every 2000 anesthetics. (The accepted estimated figure for deaths under ether anesthesia is one in 16,000 anesthesias.) Each year 10,000,000 anesthesias are given in this country. This would tend to suggest that there are 5000 monuments annually dedicated to this clinical disaster. This catastrophe is a greater killer than dreaded anterior poliomyelitis.* During the epidemic year of 1952 there were less than 4000 deaths attributed to this disease.

In one hospital** in Cleveland 15,000 anesthesias were given in the year 1951. In that institution there were fourteen cases of sudden death on the operating table during the same year. In a large general hospital in Cleveland, 26,612 surgical anesthetics were given over a three-and-one-half year period; there was an occurrence rate of 1 in 739, with a thirty-three per cent survival rate.

There seems to be little agreement or comparison in the data accumulated by various authors. This is understandable, as there are so many variables and intangible factors that must be considered. Some authors appear to make an attempt to differentiate true primary cardiac arrest on the operating table from secondary arrest on the operating table. This is not a practical differentiation at the operating table, but only at the autopsy table. The practical result is to preserve the patient's life by immediate action. Let us not quibble.

Obviously not included in these figures are the anesthetics given by the dental profession. It has been

*Salk vaccine clinically introduced in 1956.
**Personal communication.

determined that there are approximately 60,000,000 of this type each year. Intravenous anesthesia can be particularly hazardous if no provision has been made to supply additional oxygen into the trachea and alveoli. A face mask will not permit the operator to work in mouth.

Cole and Corday, in a report, estimated that in Los Angeles, California, two-hundred thirty cases of cardiac arrest occur annually.

Certainly these statistics clearly denote that it is not a rarity. Another approach to this aspect of the subject may be taken by considering the number of surgical deaths in a general hospital, comparing the percentage cardiac arrest has played. For instance, in one *700-bed hospital in 1952 there were thirty-two deaths on the surgical service, five of the thirty-two occurring from cardiac arrest. In other words, cardiac arrest as a surgical complication in this hospital accounted for $15\frac{1}{2}\%$ of the deaths. Is it a rare surgical complication?

Fatalities in the operating room each year from static electrical sparks are variously reported from twenty to less than one-hundred. Seriously compare the precautions, education, and cost of available equipment that have been given and directed to combat these two unexpected and dissimilar operating room phenomena. Once the task of eliminating explosion hazards has been accomplished, the per-

*Personal communication to the author.

sonnel will often relax and drift with the stream. Constant vigilance and education is necessary to prevent sudden cardiac stoppage.

Some statistics indicate that fifty per cent of these cardio-respiratory deaths occur in individuals in the fourth to sixth decade. Also in these decades occurs the highest operative incidence. The incidence of cessation of the heart beat is obviously increased in cardiac and lung surgery. Blalock found cardiac massage necessary in five and one-half per cent of the patients operated upon for pulmonary stenosis.

This disaster can complicate any type of operation. Nevertheless, one is impressed by the fact that it occurs rather frequently during a simple procedure for which the patient has been judged to be a good surgical risk, and often the poor-risk patient on whom we have hesitated to operate, unbelievably "sails through without mishap." Subsequently, one often wonders why one was hesitant. Could this observation mean that in the second instance everybody in the operating room was alert and a little more "on his toes"?

One author reported that thirty-seven per cent of his collected series had occurred during minor operations. Thus the catastrophic result ultimately was more injurious than the disease for which the operation was undertaken.

Patients with known cardiac conditions (provided they are not decompensated) undergo surgery as well as so-called normal patients, assuming that the anesthetic induction and the level of anesthesia are carried out wisely and that the surgeon uses skill and judgment.

The two conditions of cessation of the heart beat that confront the surgeon in the operating room are cardiac standstill and ventricular fibrillation. The odds of finding one or the other condition differ from one group of case histories to another. There are also many factors which influence either occurrence. Fortunately, cardiac standstill or asystole will be met more frequently as it is the easier of the two circumstances to treat. In some series as well as our own, ventricular fibrillation or delirium cordis is found almost as often as standstill. This could be a disturbing thought, if the hospital did not have the special equipment necessary for the treatment of ventricular fibrillation.

These sudden deaths occur in dental offices following the administration of anesthesia. They too frequently are reported in the newspapers as heart attacks. These victims become coroners' cases, and usually no organic reason for death is established at the autopsy. The dental profession is also becoming interested in preventing such occurrences.*

At one time the false impression existed that

*In May 1957, a group of 24 dentists in Cleveland, Ohio petitioned us to arrange a special two day course for them. The course was enthusiastically received.

victims of epilepsy seldom die during a major seizure, and the extreme anoxia they suffer is the expected familiar picture. In 1951 Doctors Victoroff and Fetterman approached the author with some unusual reports of death during epileptic attacks. As an autopsy revealed no cause of death, it seemed logical that in the occasional person such a degree of anoxia can develop that at times cardiac standstill or ventricular fibrillation may ensue.

By the number of references to it in the daily newspapers and weekly magazines, are we being led to believe that this tragedy is becoming commonplace? If so, would this represent progress in present day surgery and anesthesia? This is a challenge for us all seriously to contemplate. It is my considered opinion that we must do something drastic to stop the trend of events. Some have taken the view that the relative frequency has not increased when the number of operations and the magnitude of these operations is taken into consideration.

Bost reviewed the literature and reported the grand total of one-hundred seventy-eight patients subjected to massage from 1902 to 1951.

From 1946 until 1952 the pendulum of occurrence of cardiac arrest in the operating room was swinging alarmingly upward, but since that time through the unveiling and disbursal of old and new knowledge of the subject, the pendulum now appears to be definitely on the down-grade.

The average surgeon carries the thought that such a catastrophe "can never happen to me"; therefore he may neglect to apprise himself of methods to circumvent or combat this unexpected disaster. This is an entirely human reaction—just as when reading in the newspaper that a pedestrian has been struck down while crossing the street, one unconsciously says to himself "that will never happen to me." However, once it occurs, it may be too late in that particular instance, but humility will become the stepping stone to knowledge.

There is no need to frighten or allow patients to become frightened into believing that cardiac stoppage in the operating room is a common occurrence, but it is not a rarity. It will occur at least a half a dozen times each year in every good-sized general hospital, which indicates its infrequency during the careers of many present day surgeons.

VI

MECHANISM OF THE HEART BEAT

THE HUMAN HEART will beat if given the opportunity. Cardiac muscle has the inherent quality of rhythmicity. Early in the development of the chick embryo when the anlage of the heart can be distinguished, the small myotomes can be seen to have a rhythmic motion. Coordinate beats occur before neuroblasts have reached the heart.

Heart muscle is not dependent, as are skeletal muscles, upon external stimuli to initiate contractions. In short, the heart has the property of initiating impulses (rhythmicity) and spreading them through the cardiac syncytium (conductivity). The heart demonstrates this inherent quality of beating by the independent rhythm of the ventricles during complete heart block. All parts of the heart have the properties of initiating and conducting impulses. It is apparent that a gradient of rhythmicity exists from the sinus venosus to the apex.

It is well known that the isolated heart from a cold blooded species will beat for days if kept moist. The isolated heart from a warm blooded animal will continue to maintain perfect rhythmic activity for hours if perfused with oxygenated solutions. The fact that the heart will beat when completely divorced from the body indicates that the origin of the heart beat is in the musculature itself.

Kuliabko, in 1902, restored the heart beat in a series of rabbits' hearts that had been kept in an ice chest for forty-four hours. They continued to beat for three to four days. This author was also successful in restoring the heart beat for one hour in a three-month-old infant, twenty-four hours a f t e r death. In 1912, Rhomer and Robinson showed that the heart in a state of arrest retains a latent ability to function for some time.

Under normal conditions, or normal sinus rhythm, the sino-auricular node is the starting place of each excitatory process or impulse and is called the pacemaker. The impulse spreads radially through the auricles and arrives at the atrio-ventricular node when it momentarily pauses, and is then carried along the Bundle of His and spreads out to all parts of the ventricles. This auriculo-ventricular bundle is the only functional neuromuscular connection between the auricles and the ventricles. Distribution of these impulses gives rise to the pattern of the electrocardiogram. If the S-A node is put out of action, usually the A-V node can take over and call the signals. This is referred to as a shift or transfer of the pacemaker to the A-V node. The normal sinus rhythm, A-V nodal rhythm, beats originating from ectopic foci, auricular fibrillation, and ventricular tachycardia, are the ordinary mechanisms of the heart beat which interest the surgeon in the operating room. Two conditions of cardiac arrest are encountered by the surgeon, cardiac asystole and ventricular fibrillation. Life is impossible under these latter conditions.

The heart must be adapted to the needs of the body as a whole, and its automatic nature must usually lie subservient to the central nervous system. It must, at times, either speed up or slow down to adjust itself to the changes in peripheral resistance and humoral influences. Although dogs have survived the extirpation of all afferent and efferent nerve fiber connections to the heart, their survival period is limited to months, and they cannot again lead an active normal life.

There are two main paired nerve elements leading to the heart. These are the vagus nerve from the medulla and the sympathetic system from the upper region of the spinal cord. They are antagonistic in their actions. The foremost action of vagal stimulation is to slow the heart and that of sympathetic stimulation is to speed up the heart. The right vagus seems to have the greater influence, probably due to its closer association with the S-A node in the right auricle. All parts of the heart receive sympathetic innervation.

Vagus stimulation results in slowing of the atria and ventricles, decrease of vigor of atrial contractions, and dilatation of the whole heart during diastole. The tonic action of the vagus may be increased by morphine, by rise of blood pressure in the medulla, intracranial pressure, asphyxia, Bainbridge and carotid reflexes, and some other circumstances which one cannot adequately explain. This inhibitory effect can be abolished by atropine.

DEVELOPMENT OF CARDIAC STANDSTILL

Failure of the S-A node to act as a pacemaker occasionally occurs due to intensive vagal stimulation in the operating room. There may be vagal escape in which the pacemaker shifts to the A-V node. This is characterized by a slow but effective beat. If the rhythm developed by the ventricles is very slow and the blood pressure low, the beats may become feebler and weaker and finally cease. This is due to inadequate coronary blood pressure. The shift of the pacemaker cannot occur if other subsidiary centers are depressed by the anesthetic agent. The result then is cardiac standstill. Standstill can also occur from A-V block although the auricles are contracting under the stimulus of the S-A node. This is revealed in the electrocardiograms by the presence of P waves and the absence of ventricular complexes. Displacement of the pacemaker to the nodal rhythm (A-V) and bradycardia are precursors of ventricular standstill. Reid, Stephenson and Hinton state that a heart under anesthesia is as vulnerable to vagus stimulation and slowing, as a heart with a diffuse organic lesion would be without anesthesia.

Stimulation of the sympathetic nerve has the opposite effect of that produced by stimulation of the vagus nerve. An injection of adrenalin has the same effect as sympathetic stimulation. There is an increase in the heart rate and the strength of contraction is augmented. The blood pressure and the tone are increased, the size of the heart and the venous pressure decreased. Adrenalin causes the heart to increase its oxygen usage two or three times above normal.

Cold decreases the heart rate and its irritability. Heat has the opposite effect. These facts are of some importance in the resuscitation procedure and also in hypothermic investigations.

In standstill the heart will respond to artificial stimulation. After a minute or so these tissues lose their excitability to all * forms of stimuli, artificial or natural. The heart and body are in a state of anabiosis and within certain limits this excitability can be restored by massaging oxygenated blood through the coronary arteries. Thus given the opportunity its inherent quality of rhythmicity again becomes mani-

---

*Important for consideration of external defibrillation and application of a pacemaker.

fest. There are recorded cases of successful revival of the heart beat from the injection of drugs into the heart through the intact thorax. Many of us have heard of this, but few of us actually know of specific instances. However, the stimulus of the needle is thought to be the decisive factor rather than the drug. H. Bailey[1] used intracardiac injections of adrenalin in forty cases without success.

Premature contractions can occur from epicardial stimulation and from impulses originating outside the sinus node in the auricles or ventricles. If they discharge periodically there develops a paroxysmal tachycardia. The threshold for these varies with the anesthetic agent. With some agents the threshold is decreased (chloroform), with others increased (procaine). Manipulation of the heart may excite extrasystoles and disturb the blood pressure.

Ventricular paroxysmal tachycardia may lead into ventricular flutter and fibrillation. Ordinarily it is thought that in the development of ventricular fibrillation the above pattern is followed. Auricular fibrillation is compatible with life, but ventricular fibrillation is not. In auricular fibrillation the excitatory process is rapid and disorganized. At one time it was thought to be due to a contraction impulse or circuitous excitation of the myocardium around the S-A node. The A-V node is bombarded frequently, but most of these stimuli fall into its refractory period; therefore by selectivity only a few stimuli are carried down to the ventricles. The ventricles contract irregularly and at a relatively normal rate and are able to sustain a satisfactory blood pressure, while the atria display fine irregular incoordinated movements.

VENTRICULAR FIBRILLATION

Ludwig and Hoffa, in 1849, were the first to recognize ventricular fibrillation. Vulpian in 1874 named it "mouvement fibrillaire." It is called by other terms such as delirium cordis and convulsion* of the heart. There is complete incoordination of the muscle fibres (see page 40). Each fiber and fibril is contracting at its own cadence. With the advent of the newer oscillographs, it has been estimated that the rate may reach 50,000 per minute. It is the cause of sudden death from acute coronary occlusion, electrocution, hypothermic conditions, and overdoses of certain anesthetic agents. Death occurs much faster than would occur from a stab or gunshot wound of the heart or from a bullet through the brain.

Ventricular fibrillation appears to result from a condition which produces accelerating groups of ectopic repetitive discharges (coronary occlusion, electrical currents). In the former these stimuli would seem to arise in the boundary zone between ischemic and non-ischemic muscle. In over-all anox-

---

*A convulsion results in a purposeless movement of muscle.

ia and hemorrhage there is no such boundary, and cardiac standstill supervenes and is featured by pacemaker failure.

Various hypotheses have been advanced to account for the incoordinate inefficient contractions. There are two main schools of thought centered about the idea: (a) that impulses arise from centers or pacemakers; (b) that the condition is due to re-entry of impulses and circles of excitation.[2] Once this incoordinated rhythm has been established, there is an immediate and precipitous fall of blood pressure to zero, although upon observation there is a slight quivering movement of the organ. (This fall of blood pressure is illustrated in the blood pressure tracing [Figure No. 1].) There is, however, no circulation or movement of blood. This is plainly seen upon viewing the heart, for the blood in the coronary vessels remains red as the oxygen is suddenly trapped. The blood in the coronary veins does not become bluish black. When the heart undergoes failure from standstill, it is a somewhat more gradual process. In this latter instance the veins and arteries are practically the same color. The heart writhes like a mass of earth worms and gradually dilates during the fibrillary stage. As minutes progress these fibrillary movements pass from a coarse pattern to very weak imperceptible movements. If the chest is opened late, one is apt to be misled in believing that the heart has stopped in standstill. Upon the institu-

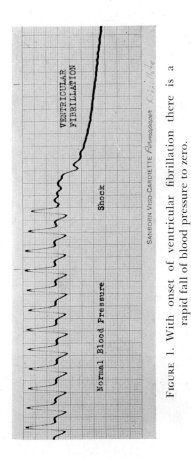

FIGURE 1. With onset of ventricular fibrillation there is a
rapid fall of blood pressure to zero.

tion of proper cardiac massage, the heart may be
seen to retrace its pattern from weak fibrillation to
coarse fibrillation. Massage of the arrested heart will
not ordinarily induce fibrillation. The stimulation
from massage will not ordinarily change a standstill
into fibrillation. Visualization of a rapid ventricular
tachycardia may at times be confused with a coarse
ventricular fibrillation. There is truly a "world" of
difference between them. Palpating the aorta, one
finds a weak pulse with the former rhythm and a collapsed pulseless aorta with the latter condition.

It seems paradoxical that the heart will at times
tolerate such injury as prolonged massage, stab
wounds, steering wheel accidents and even removal
of sections of heart muscle, yet it is so vulnerable to
occlusion of one of its coronary vessels. A small
amount[3] of oxygenated blood delivered to ischemic
muscle can reduce the destruction of heart muscle
fibers and can also reduce the incidence of ventricular fibrillation. Experiments[3] by Beck and associates
indicated that in the dog heart a back flow of 5cc. of
blood per minute protected the heart from ventricular fibrillation after coronary occlusion.

It conspicuously appears that it is only the ischemic heart which will not stand up under injury. As
a rule no permanent damage is done to the myocardium after *proper* prolonged or vigorous massage.
Minor degrees of subepicardial hemorrhage can be
seen and at times there will be electrocardiogram

changes indicative of this for a few days. These clear up entirely within a week.

It is highly advisable that the surgeon who performs heart massage have some knowledge of how to carry out proper massage. Improper technique can readily result in lacerations of the myocardium. The time and place to learn this proper technique is upon the dog's heart in the laboratory.

BIBLIOGRAPHY

1. Bailey, H.: Impending Death Under Anesthesia. *Brit. M. J.,* 2:84, 1941.
2. Wiggers, C. J.: Circulation on Health and Disease. Fifth Edition.
3. Hahn, R. S.; Kim, M.; Beck, C. S.: Revascularization of the Heart. *Am. Heart J.,* 44:472, 1952.

VII

OXYGEN AND THE BRAIN

THE MOST HIGHLY developed organ in the human body, the brain, is the most vulnerable to lack of oxygen. The existence of anoxia for a length of time somewhere between three to five minutes results in irreversible damage. The pathologic physiology is considered a severe state of cerebral edema. The newest areas of the brain phylogenetically are the most rapidly injured, so that higher central nervous system functions, such as speaking, thinking, and remembering, are most likely to be permanently impaired by periods of anoxia greater than three to five minutes. It is estimated* that the basal ganglia[1] of the brain will withstand a lack of oxygen for a length of time from twenty to thirty minutes.**

The vulnerability of the cerebral cortical cells to complete lack of oxygen for more than three to five minutes at normal temperatures is the foremost problem in resuscitation procedures. Not all parts of the brain are equally sensitive to complete or partial

---

*Wiggers.

**At ordinary room temperature.

oxygen deprivation. Consciousness is usually lost within forty-five seconds.

The supply of oxygen to the brain is dependent upon the following factors, which are variable: the efficiency of the lungs, the efficiency of the heart as a pump, the condition of the blood and blood vessels, the integrity of the sino-aortic reflexes, and last but not least—the composition of the inspired respiratory gases.

The cause of death in patients some twelve to forty-eight hours after an effective circulation has been restored by resuscitative methods is due to cerebral edema. In these cases the arbitrary time limitation has been exceeded, yet often no difficulty is experienced in restoring the heart beat.

The effects of anoxia on the brain may be twofold: (1) Lessened oxygen tension in the arterial blood. (2) Followed by a secondary vasomotor disturbance or ischemia. The ischemia may manifest itself by dilatation and engorgement of vessels or by spasm or compression. In resuscitation this second factor may be the more difficult to treat and it can be the more devastating, as a vicious circle is set up depriving the vulnerable cells of oxygen. Any degree of cerebral edema, caused by drugs, alcohol, anoxemia may be the starting point on this predicated circle. In severe anemias the engorgement factor does not take place. (See L. Hill, pg. 47.)

The author has carried out the following experiments upon one hundred forty mongrel dogs. The dogs had been newly acquired and had not been under observation or study (possible similiarity to some clinical elective operations.) A pair of dogs was operated upon under sterile conditions on separate days. Ether anesthesia in a closed system was used. In one dog the oxygen system was broken down (ventricular fibrillation) for two minutes and then the animal was resuscitated.

In the other, the oxygen system was seriously impaired for five to six minutes and then completely disrupted for two minutes. The technic used was: clamping the intratrachial tube and observing the heart become cyanotic and dilated and its beat become feebler and feebler until it ceased. This usually took about 5 to 6 minutes. During the last agonal beats (30 seconds to 60 seconds) no palpable heart beat could be noted in the thoracic aorta. Following standstill nothing was done for two minutes, and then resuscitation was carried out.

The animals were observed twenty-four hours later. The dogs whose oxygen system was disrupted for two minutes showed complete recovery in all seventy instances. They would eat, drink, wag their tails, and run about as if nothing had happened.

In the other series of dogs, many diversified results were observed. If it could be said that a pattern evolved, it would be that this would represent a sick dog who was oblivious to his surroundings and showed stiffness and loss of function of his hind legs. However, a great many results were observed, ranging from no noticeable untoward effects, to death during the night. In the individual dog one is dealing with many variables; the only controlled factor was the length of time of the disruption of the oxygen system. The same variables are at work in the human during a moderately prolonged period of anoxia and the same diversity of results are reported.

There are many variables that influence this so-called "time limitation" in which we are all vitally interested. With this fact in mind, it is essential that pessimism should not prevail, and the surgeon should always initiate the resuscitation procedure within reasonable time limits. Usually no one person in the operating room is quite sure of the exact time of cardiac arrest. Anxiety masks a correct estimation of time. This is understandable if previous planning has not been initiated.

Fundamentally, the metabolism or oxygen needs of individuals vary. For instance, some persons can tolerate much higher altitudes* than others before black-out supervenes. The reactions of the cardio-vascular system to progressively diminishing oxygen shows kaleidoscopic individual[2] variation.

Body temperature is one determining factor in metabolism. Within reasonable ranges, metabolism is thought to vary seven per cent for each degree of change. This no doubt accounts for incredible re-ports of complete recovery after drowning. It was found, in looking up[2b] some of these reports, that these persons had fallen through ice. The war records and Dachau experiments indicated that submersion in icy waters was the fastest means of bringing down the body temperatures.

Experiments[2a] with small animals tend to indi-cate that they can be protected from low concentra-tion of oxygen by the administration of large doses of adrenal cortex. These animals withstood the equivalent of three times the altitude of the control animals.

The metabolic pattern of each person varies and is also related to the coenzyme system of cellular

---

*Natives of Peru play tournament soccer at an elevation of 15,000 feet. In 1875 three Frenchman ascended to 27,900 feet in a balloon. When the balloon reached the ground, only one was alive.

oxidation. It obviously includes inherited characteristics that are individualistic and distinctive. Such
oxidation[1] does not occur through direct combination of organic substances with molecular oxygen; it
is accomplished through complex oxidation—reduction systems, the nature of which still remains somewhat confused. The site and function of genetotroph-
ic blocks may be determined by genetic factors and
is interwoven with the coenzyme oxidative system.
If shock or hypoxia is pronounced, there is a breakdown of the co-enzyme system. A good pre-operative
nutritional state is the best preventive measure
against a breakdown of the co-enzyme system, if any
metabolism is to be maintained in an hypoxic or
anoxic condition.

In many instances of cardiac arrest there may be
a certain degree of anesthetic cerebral hypoxia preceding the actual heart stoppage. Cerebral hypoxia
can occur through narcotic depression of the respiratory center and vasomotor center. This fact has a
definite influence upon the safe time limitation. In
this instance it would be incorrect to assume that the
brain was deficient in oxygen only from time of cessation. A certain and definite degree of cerebral injury had taken place preceding the anoxia of arrest.

Age is a factor to take into consideration. Young
persons, especially newborn infants, tolerate cerebral
anoxia more satisfactorily than the old. Heinwich refers to recent experiments which indicate that the
newborn, in comparison to the adult, processes an

extra-ordinary resistance to anoxia. It appears that those individuals who have withstood repeated attacks of syncope related to the Stokes-Adams syndrome and those with chronic emphysema can withstand a lack of oxygen and an accumulation of carbon dioxide for a slightly longer time. It is referred to as acclimatization.

Considerable research has been done in an attempt to improve the circulation of the brain. It has been found that in the healthy individual with a normal circulatory system, little can be done[3] to increase or speed up cerebral circulation. Under ordinary circumstances it remains remarkably constant. Changes in position or the use of vasodilator drugs have little if any effect. However, the inhalation of five to seven per cent carbon dioxide can increase cerebral blood flow[3,4,5], seventy-five per cent. This action is thought to be due to the acidosis produced. The antianoxic action of carbon dioxide has been recognized for a long time. This should be remembered in those patients in whom it is desirable to speed up the cerebral circulation. The administration of oxygen in concentration above room air may cause a slight constriction of cerebral vessels. These physiologic findings apply to the normally functioning circulatory system which is not under the influence of anesthetic drugs. In cardiac arrest, with its accompanying disruption of the circulatory system, the 10 degree Trendelenburg position is beneficial. This results in improvement of cerebral[6] circulation.

Under these abnormal conditions oxygen concentrations higher than room air are also of tremendous importance.

We know that certain organs (such as the heart and brain) are able to extract an unusually high amount of oxygen from the blood. In some instances the heart* is virtually able to wring out practically all of the oxygen from the circulating blood. The normal cerebral blood flow represents approximately fourteen per cent of the total cardiac output. Normally the brain extracts considerably more oxygen from the blood flowing through it than does either the liver or kidney. Thus the brain, an organ of only 1400^3 grams, accounts for twenty-two per cent of the total oxygen consumption of the body. In heart failure, blood flow can be reduced forty per cent, yet greatly increased oxygen extraction results in only thirteen per cent decrease in cerebral oxygen con-the body is modified[1,4], regionally, being increased sumption. During progressive hypoxia, blood flow in through the brain and coronary vessels by vasodilatation and decreased through the skin by vaso-constriction.

The above information tends to clarify the observation that constant blood pressures sustained around 50 mm. of mercury will help keep these high-

---

*There are other compensatory mechanisms which strive to make up for the scarcity of oxygen, and they may succeed in restoring functions to near normal.

er centers viable during a period of manual massage. Hill[8], in 1899, pointed out that the brain can continue its functions with a greatly reduced blood supply by referring to animal experiments and to the lack of marked cerebral symptoms in those patients with advanced pernicious anemia.

BIBLIOGRAPHY

1. Wiggers, C. J.: Circulation in Health and Disease. Fifth Edition.
2. Titrud, L. A.; Haymaker, W.: Cerebral Anoxia From High Altitude Asphyxiation. *Arch. Neurol. & Psychiat., 57*:397, 1947.
2a. Thorne, G. W., *et al.*: Adrenal Cortex High Altitude Relationship. *Endocrinology, 36*:381, 1945.
2b. Hosler, R.: Cardiac Arrest in the Operating Room. *J. Am. Nurse Anesth., 20*:18, 1952.
3. Scheinberg, P.; Jayne, H. W.: Factors Influencing Cerebral Blood Flow and Metabolism. *Circulation, 5*:225, 1952.
4. Kety, S. S.; Schmidt, C. F.: Effects of Altered Arterial Tensions of Carbon Dioxide and Oxygen on Cerebral Blood Flow. *J. Clin. Investigation, 27*:500, 1948.
5. Gibbs, F. A.; Maxwell, H.; Gibbs, E. L.: *Arch. Neurol. & Psychiat., 57*:137, 1947.
6. Cole, F.: Head Lowering in the Treatment of Hypotension. *J.A.M.A., 150*:273, 1952.
7. Loman and Myerson: Circulation of Brain and Face. *Arch. Neurol. & Psychiat., 57*:94, 1947.
8. Hill, L.: Albutt System of Medicine. Vol. 8, p. 262, 1899.

VIII

ETIOLOGY

IN SOME PATIENTS the specific cause of cardiac arrest is entirely clear and can be pin-pointed. In other instances this is not the case; it may be the result of a chain of circumstances, and somewhere along this chain a link is broken which precipitates this disaster.

In taking into consideration the etiological factors in this situation, almost without exception, the cause of cardiac arrest ultimately resolves itself into a lack of oxygen in the vital tissues with an accumulation of carbon dioxide. Anoxia constitutes one of the gravest hazards to the surgical patient. The immediate effect on the brain and myocardium are the most serious. A breakdown in the oxygen system occurs. This lack of oxygen is the result of either impaired ventilation or impaired circulation, the former occurring more frequently. Hypoxia may occur, either by hypoventilation or blood loss. At times this may occur insidiously or may be sudden. It is typical of severe hypoxia that when respiration and circulation fail, they fail suddenly. This breakdown of the oxygen system may be transitory and is therefore reversible within a certain time requirement.

The cardiorespiratory system is referred to in presenting this subject in the simplified term—the oxygen system. The heart and lungs may fail to function simultaneously or one may fail before the other. It is unimportant which fails first. They cannot function separately. Life is a continuous process of oxygenation. To the cell, life, oxygen, and metabolism are synonomous.

Physiology texts present the respiratory system and the cardiovascular system in separate chapters. Respiration and circulation are often thought of as individual entities. The functions of the heart and lungs are so interdependent that when one fails, failure of the other will follow shortly.

What do we mean by re-establishing the oxygen system? In simple, understandable terms we mean performing three functions:

First, get oxygen into the lungs.

Second, have enough available hemoglobin to transport the oxygen.

Finally, provide a dynamic pump to propel the oxygenated hemoglobin to the brain and other organs in order that they will remain viable. The heart remains a satisfactory hydro-dynamic pump, provided the surgeon gets his hand upon it and carries out purposeful manual massage.

PREDISPOSING FACTORS CONTRIBUTING TO CARDIAC ARREST PRIOR TO THE OPERATION INCLUDE:

1. Insufficient preoperative dosage of atropine.
2. Multiplicity and over-dosage of preanesthetic drugs.
3. Excessive administration of digitalis, quinidine, and papaverine, etc.
4. Underlying cardiac disease.
5. Decreased vital capacity. ⎫
6. Poor cardiac filling. ⎬ Position of patient
7. Anemia.
8. Poor state of nutrition.
9. Anxiety.
   Pheochromocytoma
10. Shock.
11. Excessive speed of induction of anesthetic agents.
12. Errors of judgment.
13. Abnormally elevated body temperature.
14. Racial predisposition.

Many of the above factors are self-explanatory.

DRUGS

Atropine is a valuable drug in protecting the heart from the efferent reflexes that may be instituted through the vagus nerve—that is the vago-vagal reflex and the carotid reflex. The vago-vagal reflex produces an overabundance of acetylcholine (Figs. 2 and 3). The heart is sensitive to acetylcholine. These afferent reflexes can be created readily in vago-tonic individuals in the nasopharynx, region of ocular orbit, esophagus, trachea, bronchial tree, stomach, gallbladder, intestinal mesenteries, rectum, and bladder. Sloan, as well as Starling, demonstrated in animals that the vago-vagal reflex will only cause cardiac stoppage in the presence of definite hypoxia. It is well to give a patient of average size a pre-operative dosage of at least 1/100 grain of atropine to inhibit vagal activity. If the patient is unduly delayed before the anesthetic is started, it is desirable to have it repeated. During a long anesthetic it can be repeated intravenously every two hours if a sinus bradycardia appears.

The frequent practice of giving several drugs during the preanesthetic period and during the induction is often detrimental* and may cause cerebral depression. The administration of a multiplicity of drugs is highly inadvisable. It is well known that certain individuals have drug idiosyncrasies, and in the occasional individual who has had five or six drugs the offending agent may be masked or compounded. Only a few individuals fall into this category, as in

---

*Flagg has referred to this as experimental pharmacology moving into the operating room.

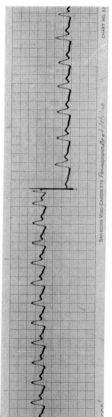

FIGURE 2. The effect of acetylcholine which is similar to a vagus response. The blood pressure at onset was 160/115. There is an obvious slowing of the pulse rate decline of blood pressure to 95/40.

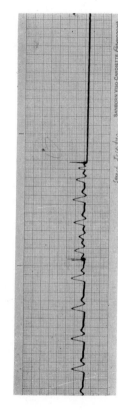

FIGURE 3. After the second injection of acetylcholine the heart stops in standstill.

the majority of instances the difficulty is overdosage.

Patients who have received generous and prolonged dosages of the rawolfia and the chlorpromazine group of medicaments must receive careful evaluation and attention, otherwise unpredictable circulatory disturbances may occur. The same is true of cortisone. We are all familiar with its present wide usage, particularly in arthritic conditions. Withdrawal of this drug may assign the individual to the jeopardy of Pseudo-Addison's disease. Massive citrated blood transfusions can interfere with the normal clotting mechanisms, and at the same time the excessive amount of citrate can upset the important calcium potassium ion relationship. This relationship assumes more importance to a patient undergoing an anesthesia, as any change in the pH of the blood or change in oxygen and carbon dioxide content of the blood will change or upset this ionic relationship.

Elective cardiac arrest is now being carried out for intracardiac surgery. Potassium citrate is injected at the root of the aorta, and the drug is directed into the coronary channels by back pressure. The heart is quiescent and the systemic circulation is carried on with an extra corporoeal heart-lung oxygenator and pump. This would tend to focus attention on the role of the relationship of the blood electrolytes as a causative factor of arrest.

The heavily pre-medicated patient is usually pleased with the anesthetic and enjoys the knowledge that he does not remember leaving his room. The surgeon, in general, prefers the plane of anesthesia as he can complete his abdominal surgery without fighting the intestines. However, if disaster overtakes one patient the result is complete and irreparable. Too often the incriminating expression has been used: "The patient was overdrugged and underoxygenated."

Overdosages of digitalis, quinidine and paverine act like poisons or toxins to the myocardium and interfere with the metabolism of the heart. Inhibition of potassium ion transfer is believed to take place in cardiac standstill from digitalis intoxication.

CARDIAC DISEASE

Cardiac disease requires little explanation. Hearts with coronary disease already may have a reduction of oxygenated blood and any additional degree of anoxia could be disastrous.

Sudden fluctuations of blood pressure and arterial oxygen saturations might occasionally and conceivably produce an electrically[1] and unstable heart with subsequent sudden mechanism death.

VITAL CAPACITY

Normal individuals have a generous reserve of vital capacity. In the average elective operation too little attention is devoted to this subject. A reduction of vital capacity must be carefully considered and evaluated. It can be the result of pulmonary disease, emphysema, hemorrhage in the lung, pressure pneumothorax, pulmonary edema, and similar conditions. Pulmonary edema may suddenly occur in the course of an operation. This has been noted during cardiac surgery. It may clear up as quickly as it appears if proper measures are immediately put into operation. Instances have been reported of patients undergoing surgery who have been known to have a low or border-line vital capacity, who have been placed in jeopardy of cardiac arrest by the use of an endotracheal aspiration catheter for an excessively long period. The catheter also removed too great an amount of oxygen over too long a period, thus pushing the patient into a severe degree of anoxic hypoxia.

A full 50 per cent of the chances for survival can be deprived the patient during an operation or during this emergency if the endotracheal tube is improperly placed into a mainstem bronchus. Such an error permits utilization of only one lung, rendering the other lung useless.

POSITION OF THE PATIENT

The position of the patient on the operating table can and does influence his vital capacity. A person can breath more easily flat on his back with the head and shoulders slightly elevated. Any other position tends to impair the vital capacity to varying degrees. As a rule during an elective operation the patient has such a reserve that ordinary changes of position are relatively unimportant. The deep Trendelenburg position in an obese patient may cause a dangerous reduction of vital capacity. The heavy abdominal organs push up the diaphram and encroach upon the lungs, reducing his vital capacity by one-third. At the same time this extreme position lends itself to an increase of carbon dioxide tension in the blood. A considerable reduction in vital capacity occurs in the Kraske position, while a lesser degree results from the lateral or Simms position.

A profound change in blood pressure can occur when any patient is turned on the operating table. Ether, the procaine group and spinal anesthesia relax the peripheral vascular system in the extremities, resulting in a pooling* of the circulating volume of blood. Any change in position should be gradual.

CARDIAC FILLING

Poor cardiac filling with concomitant reduction of cardiac output may result from the position of the patient during an operative procedure. This is an important consideration in those operations in which the patient is in a sitting position—for instance, in certain brain operations and during many so-called minor nose and throat operative procedures. There is

---

*Only 11% of the total blood volume is normally within the arterial portion of the circulatory system.

a pooling of blood in the extremities and splanchnic area with an incomplete return of blood to the heart. As the heart fills incompletely, in time there is a breakdown of the mechanism sustaining blood pressure, and suddenly the patient may be in a dangerous state. Sudden reduction of intra-abdominal pressure from delivery of large tumors, cysts, multiple pregnancies, rapid catheterization of an overdistended urinary bladder, and similar procedures, may have this end result. Without an adequate return of blood to the heart, the output in turn will be correspondingly reduced. Sudden hemorrhage has in part the same effect. A sudden change from the lithotomy position after a prolonged procedure results in a pooling of the blood in the extended lower extremities.

Our group[2] has pointed out that the greatest hazard in most otolaryngological operations is the sitting position. Gradually the old straight backed stationary chair has been replaced by tilt reclining chairs.

ANEMIA

Anemia may contribute to cardiac arrest under anesthesia by increasing the degree of hypoxia. This is referred to as an anemic hypoxia as distinct from anoxic hypoxia. A stagnant type of hypoxia occurs during the failure of the circulation. A state of hypoxia increases the sensitivity of the heart to acetylcholine as well as epenephrine. An inhibitor to this substance, cholinesterase, is thought to be present on the surface of the red blood cells. It follows, if during surgery vago-vagal reflexes are initiated, acetylcholine is produced in the myocardial fibers at their end plates. Thus, if the cardiac sensitivity to acetylcholine has been increased (hypoxia, or if the cholinesterase is decreased) the heart will respond by slowing and at times proceeding to complete standstill (vagus influence). An inadequate volume of circulating blood results in anemic hypoxia. It is impossible, even with the best anesthetic equipment, to blow oxygen through an empty arteriovenous system. An anemic patient can become sub-oxygenated in a hurry without necessarily showing a profound degree of cyanosis.

NUTRITION

For any operation the patient must be in the best state of nutrition possible under the prevailing circumstances. Laboratory study should indicate adequate protein and glycogen reserves. The electrolytic state should be investigated. This is particularly important in the two extremes of life. Under conditions of shock the administration of vitamins (particularly thiamine) has been found of great value in the preservation of tissue coenzymes in hypoxic conditions.

ANXIETY

Anxiety and fear can result in an overdose of

adrenalin of endogenous origin. Although death is an extremely rare result of this condition, it has been reported by Cannon[3] and others to lead to death from ventricular fibrillation.

Have persons actually been frightened to death? Yes, and the usual mode of death is by ventricular fibrillation. Of course this is a rarity. The pattern has been produced in normal animals by the injection of epinephrine. This has been enhanced when the animals are anesthetized with cyclopropane or chloroform. This no doubt occurs in apprehensive humans.

SHOCK

A patient who is brought to the operating room in a degree of shock is obviously a poor anesthetic risk.

SPEED OF INDUCTION

Rapid induction of the anesthesia is a predisposing cause of cardiac arrest. This, fundamentally, is over-dosage. It is readily accomplished by the intravenous route.

ERRORS

Errors in judgment are rare, but their forms can cover an amazingly large area. Among the most common are such simple mistakes as the mis-labeling of gaseous anesthetic cylinders and the failure to change exhausted oxygen cylinders in closed type anesthetic machines. Failure to make frequent changes of soda lime. Failure of the anesthetist to remain at the head of the patient.

TEMPERATURE

Abnormally high body temperatures result in an increased consumption of oxygen by the patient. Under anesthesia, great care must be exercised to avoid a serious state of hypoxia. It has been found by Potts that moderate cooling of blue babies during the course of a long cardiac operation is a safeguard against cardiac collapse on the operating table.

Each rise or fall of one degree Fahrenheit from the normal of 98.6 degrees results in a change of metabolism of approximately seven percent. This applies for ordinary changes of body temperatures. The oxygen consumption follows a similar curve as that of metabolism, therefore it can be readily seen that an elevation of temperature could account for a twenty to twenty-five per cent increase in oxygen consumption.

During procedures under hypothermic conditions, as the temperature falls below eighty degrees, the threshold for ventricular fibrillation of the heart decreases to such an extent that at times a neglible stimulus may precipitate fibrillation.

RACIAL PREDISPOSITION

General statistics indicate that the darker races

are more predisposed to suffer cardiac arrest during anesthesia than the white race. The only logical explanation seems to be that cyanosis is harder to detect due to the pigmentation of their skin.

OTHER PREDISPOSING FACTORS POSSIBLY PRESENT DURING THE OPERATION

1. Duration of the operation.
2. Hypoxia enhances excitability of the ventricles.
3. Reflex stimulation under light anesthesia.
4. Torsion of the heart, etc.
5. Anesthetic agents. (Overdosage is common and self-explanatory.)
6. Respiratory tract and tracheal obstruction.
7. Excessive accumulation of carbon dioxide in the tissues in spite of good oxygenation.
8. Shock.
9. Apathy of anesthetist and surgical attendants.
10. Air embolism.

DURATION OF OPERATION

Factors in the duration of the operation are: length of operation and length of anesthesia.

In this era of surgery, speed is not the measure of a surgeon. However, if an operation can be done with dispatch in two hours and instead four hours are consumed, it is obvious that each cell in the body has been subjected to twice as much anesthetic drug, respiratory and cardio-vascular disturbance. This extra toll may be found excessive. The length of the operation is especially important in the young and the older age groups.

HYPOXIA

Hypoxia enhances the excitability of the ventricles and leads to premature beats and, finally, abnormal rhythms such as ventricular tachycardia which can go on to ventricular fibrillation.

The pattern is ventricular extra systoles, followed by runs of extra systoles, then ventricular tachycardia, ventricular flutter, and finally ventricular fibrillation. The pattern is reversible up to and including ventricular flutter, but it is extremely rare to have ventricular fibrillation spontaneously revert to a coordinated beat.

Any arrhythmia originating in the ventricles can be serious; while those which have their origin in the auricles are relatively innocuous.

REFLEX STIMULATION

Reflex stimulation under light anesthesia was thought to be a factor in one series. Sixty-six per cent of the cases of cardiac standstill and ninety-one per cent of the cases of ventricular fibrillation appeared during those periods when anesthesia was at its lightest stage. Rough handling of tissues and organs is to be deplored.

MANIPULATION OF THE HEART

Torsion and manipulation of the heart have caused arrest by creating various unfavorable conditions. Manipulation of the organ parallel to its long axis seems to cause the least disturbance. It is possible to angulate the heart so that the thinner veins (vena cavae) are compressed with the result that the chambers of the heart are poorly filled. Thus, there is created poor cardiac output and low ineffectual coronary pressure. It is also possible to compress a major coronary vessel unknowingly and have it followed by ventricular fibrillation. Surface stimulation can also cause a definite disturbance of rhythm. Although rare, it is possible to stimulate the surface of the heart with a needle or by other means and place the heart in ventricular fibrillation. This can happen* only if stimulation occurs during the split second of a certain phase of diastole. Often the surgeon is so intent upon his task that he does not notice the above train of events. It is wise and efficacious for one of the members of the team, or the anesthetist, immediately to call a halt and ask for a period of rest until conditions improve or return to normal.

---

*Beck states that he has never seen this happen in the laboratory or operating room.

ANESTHETIC* AGENTS

In considering anesthetic agents, the first step is to choose wisely, and if in any doubt, to employ the one with which the anesthetist is the most familiar. Cardiac arrest has occurred and can occur with any of the common agents. It seldom occurs in the proper state of surgical anesthesia, but it is prone to occur under light or deep anesthesia of various degrees. The effect of anesthetics on the individual heart cannot be predicted. It is well known that those persons suffering from cardiac ailments or hypertension do better with a combination of ether and nitrous oxide, or ether alone. Ether has little effect on the heart. Persons with considerable elevation of blood pressure do not do well under spinal anesthesia. Cyclopropane, chloroform, and ethyl chloride sensitize the heart to epinephrine and the heart is irritable when handled or manipulated. Overdosage of chloroform may result in myocardial depression or superimposed anoxia. Cyclopropane increases the irritability of the heart, but causes little myocardial depression. The margin of safety with cyclopropane and chloroform in many hands is small.

Sodium pentothal** possesses certain characteristics that are disadvantageous. It appears that this

---

*Oliver Wendell Holmes applied this name to the state produced by ether in the hands of Morton.
**Paulson, J. A.: Thiopental Sodium and Ether Anesth. *J.A.M.A.*, *150*:983, 1952.

agent is a potent respiratory depressant as well as a histotoxic agent. The combination of curare and pentothal must be used judiciously and intelligently. Thiopental should not be used with less than fifty per cent oxygen. It can be a myocardial depressant with associated hypoxia. Certain people question whether or not this group of intravenous agents can be classified as true anesthetic agents. Curare will cause an increase in bronchial secretions. Curare—like drugs may stop respiration. This latter statement has been known since the discovery of South America. Cocaine must be used intelligently.

Doses of more than 200 milligrams of procaine should not be used. Procaine has a depressant effect upon the heart and can stimulate the brain to convulsions. It depresses the myocardium and conduction system.

When multiple anesthetic agents are used, there is great individual difficulty in judging a correct dose. Never permit hypoxia and hypercapnia to masquerade as anesthesia.

Let us consider the unfortunate events in a *hypothetical* tonsil operation under local anesthesia. The patient is a so-called perfect specimen in the prime of life, who may or may not have had any preoperative medication. He is in a sitting position. He may be emotionally upset. The area is infiltrated with two per cent procaine (1 per cent is preferred).

Shortly thereafter, the patient becomes pale, clammy, and has a sinister bradycardia. This is the effect of an overdose of the agent and it may be quickly followed by sudden cardiovascular collapse and death. What is the mechanism of this sudden death?

It is felt that this is the effect of a high concentration of procaine (transitory overdosage) in the blood stream and not hypersensitivity. This drug quickly reaches the heart. Its effect on the heart is to relax its tone and cause a series of weak beats. Now, if the cardiac filling is also poor due to position and peripheral vascular collapse, the coronary pressure—within a dozen or so beats—can become ineffectual. Cardiac arrest quickly supervenes.

Briefly, what should the alert surgeon attempt to do in such a situation? Provided the patient is not yet pulseless, he should be placed in such a position that he is practically standing on his head. This will give him a quick matched transfusion of 600 to 700 cc. of whole blood which has been stagnant in the dependent parts. Next, the respiration must be maintained by mechanical methods. These maneuvers may be enough to prevent the termination in cardiac arrest, as within a few minutes, this transitory overdosage will have a chance to be eliminated and detoxified. If cessation of the heart beat has occurred, the above measures are carried out and without hesitation the chest is boldly opened and cardiac massage instituted.

TRACHEAL OBSTRUCTION

Respiratory or tracheal obstruction may result from obstructed airways, tumors, cysts, and abscesses in the neck, angioneurotic edema, Ludwig's angina, bilateral injury to the recurrent nerves, tracheal collapse, foreign bodies and bronchospasm, to name only a portion of the possibilities. Aspiration of vomitus is the serious offender in the operating room. This is prone to occur during emergency operations, during recovery from anesthesia, and during childbirth. Statistics concerning the latter are somewhat alarming, as usually it is preventable.

The English Ministry of Health[4] recently published the number of deaths occurring as a result of anesthesia. The commonest single cause of death was the inhalation of vomitus.

CARBON DIOXIDE

In the laboratory, it has been found that in some animals it has not been possible to bring the heart "out" of fibrillation in spite of perfect oxygenation, due to the fact that there has been an accumulation of carbon dioxide in the tissues. This occurs because the soda lime in the closed type of anesthetic machine has lost its absorptive ability. After substituting new soda lime, these same hearts can readily be brought out of ventricular fibrillation by the usual method.

Pulmonary fibrosis and emphysema as well as some form of hypoventilation result in marked ventilatory impairment resulting in carbon dioxide retention. Occasionally these patients become comatose without apparent reason. As the carbon dioxide tension rises to figures between twenty and thirty per cent, its narcotic effect becomes manifest. Perplexing and undesirable responses noted by the anesthetist may be the insidious effect of carbon dioxide retention. The knowledge that carbon dioxide is much more depressing than such anesthetics as ethylene and nitrous oxide should prevent any consideration of using it to resuscitate unless it be necessary.

An unprecedented rise of the potassium level in the blood stream may occur at the end of a prolonged operation upon washing out the carbon dioxide accumulation. It is at this moment that cardiac arrest may occur.

MISCELLANEOUS FACTORS

Of interest is the fact that Sarnoff has been able to produce pulmonary edema and cardiac arrest in animals within a few seconds after the injection of fibrin into the Cisterna Magnum. Other factors may be: Apathy of anesthetist and surgical attendants; air embolism; shock developing during the operation, rupture of trachea from intubation, and others which are numerous, but not of frequent occurrence.

Another contributing factor is the fact that a mild degree of additional hypoxia may develop following nitrous oxide anesthesia when the patient is allowed to breathe room air. This gas[5] given off in the alveoli dilutes the air coming in, and the first, ten minutes there may be a fall of the oxygen arterial tension of ten per cent. Additional oxygen may be necessary.

Shock may develop due to a hypotension of pharmacological origin. It may also develop from hidden blood loss.

BIBLIOGRAPHY

1. Brofman, B., *et al*: Electrical Instability of Heart Circ., *13*:161, 1956.
2. Hosler, R.: Cardiac Arrest from the Otolaryngologist's Viewpoint. *A.M.A. Arch. Oto.*, 57:371, 1953.
3. Cannon, W.: Voodoo Death. *Am. Anthropologist, 44:* 169, 1942.
4. English Ministry of Health Report: *Anesthesia, 2:* 194, 1956.
5. Fink, B. R., *Anesthesiology, 16:*511, 1955.

IX

PREVENTIVE MEASURES

THE BEST TREATMENT for this condition is prevention. Planning for such an eventuality is one of the best ways to avert it. The planning must be on an individual plane and also on an institutional plane, if better results are to be obtained. Preparation and education will save lives and time-consuming indecisions.

The self-contained attitude that this incident will not happen to one is dangerous and unfortunate. Once it strikes, the individual and institution acquire humility forthwith. This humility is the offspring of knowledge.

Hospital drill teams should be organized. The knowledge of special instruments and their whereabouts should be learned. If death under anesthesia is imminent, there should be a method for instantly alerting a resuscitation team. False alarms should be relished.

Pre-operatively the skillful anesthetist must evaluate each patient as to the type of anesthesia and the requirements of the operation. He must assess the emotional characteristics and attempt to have the patient arrive in the operating room with a minimal amount of fear. The hall and operating floor should not sound like a boiler factory. With these fundamental requisites taken care of, the anesthetist can avoid many of the precipitating factors. The intangible factor of experience is always present.

Pre-operative evaluation of the history of symptoms of orthopnea, shortness of breath, and precordial pain may prevent the development of this operating room disaster. Definitely abnormal blood pressures and electrocardiograms can be a premonitory sign. There is danger in administering almost any type of anesthesia to a person under the influence of alcohol. The respiratory center may be significantly depressed from the alcohol alone and the addition of further depressant drugs can lead to anoxia and respiratory acidosis. There is the additional hazard of the aspiration of vomitus.

Whether or not the patient is anemic, the expectation of the loss of blood must be considered pre-operatively. Hemoglobin values below seventy per cent must be corrected. An optimal nutritional state is desirable. A good glycogen store is necessary for a normally functioning heart. It is advisable to have all sources of infection under control, especially those that produce tracheo-bronchial secretions. Postural drainage may be necessary before anesthesia. These particular persons should be lightly premedicated. Hypoprotenemia or any deficit of fluid balance should be investigated and corrected.

Anesthetic and preanesthetic drugs can be potent factors. A death from anesthesia excites much comment from the laity, while a direct surgical complication will create less discussion. We are careful with regard to the multiplicity of anesthetic drugs and in this respect may be considered old-fashioned. (However, we do not recommend dictating the procedure to a competent anesthetist.) The pre-operative requisites of each surgical candidate should be individualized. Synergisms may occur which are little understood. A small dose of barbiturate is given on the night before the elective surgery. If local anesthesia is to be used, the barbiturate is repeated in the morning, as it increases the tolerance to a toxic reaction from procaine. The toxic excitatory phase of the procaine group can be antagonized by the barbiturates. If the rate of absorption exceeds the rate of detoxification, the concentration in the blood stream mounts. When these drugs are injected into a mucous membrane, it can be absorbed almost as quickly as if it were administered intravenously, since the mucous membrane has such an abundant blood supply. This may quickly proceed to toxic blood levels and rapidly jeopardize a surgeon's practice. Children should seldom receive barbiturates.

Morphine sulfate* (gr. 1/6) and atropine sulfate* (gr. 1/100) are given subcutaneously at least

---

*Average size adult.

one-half hour before the operative procedure. In the opinion of some authors, comparable doses of demerol and morphine have the same inhibiting effect upon the respiratory center; they also have equal tendencies to lead to addiction. Morphine produces more tendency towards periods of nausea, but it is distinctly superior in its characteristics of suppressing the cough reflex.

Atropine is given to inhibit vagal action. It is recommended in small children and during local and general tonsillectomies. A moderately rapid heart action is perferred to a bradycardia. Atropine and scopolamine have similar actions; however, atropine has more of a cardiac protective mechanism, while scopolamine has more of a central hypnotic effect. During a long procedure or if the preanesthetic drug has been given an unusually long time in advance, atropine should be repeated intravenously. This is an invaluable drug in the face of a degree of cyanosis, sinister and sudden bradycardia, and hypotension without excessive blood loss. If during surgery a patient shows bradycardia, AV dissociation or AV nodal rhythm, he should immediately receive additional intravenous atropine. The cardiac protective effect of atropine when given intravenously is thought to last from twenty-five to forty-five minutes.

An operation on the patient who has suffered a head injury should be postponed if possible. If he is drowsy and depressed the small dose of morphine may be the precipitating factor which results in a breakdown of the oxygen system.

Persons with heart disease should be re-evaluated before operation. However there is no heart disease which would contra-indicate a life saving surgical operation.

The following remarks relating to basal anesthesia are well known generalities. Rapid induction should not be undertaken. The surgical team should not "push" the anesthetist. Ether anesthesia is the choice in cardiacs and hypertensives. Cyclopropane is contra-indicated in patients with pre-operative cardiac arrhythmias. Adrenalin should not be given with cyclopropane or to patients with hypertension. Epinephrine causes the general rate of oxidation of all tissues to increase; therefore there is a greater need for oxygen. This need is hard to accommodate in the myocardium which is jeopardized by coronary sclerosis. An irritable heart or one under the influence of an anesthetic may be the seat of sudden precipitation of ventricular fibrillation by this additional action of epinephrine. Those individuals with known coronary disease are prone to have difficulties if a high degree of hypoxia is present during the induction. In the course of induction, the alveolar concentration of oxygen is at its lowest level of the entire anesthetic period; breath holding, coughing and laryngo-spasm should be averted.

We are not familiar with the use of chloroform.

Intravenous procaine is not recommended for routine thoracic surgery. A vasopressor substance must be given to combat hypotension with the introduction of the anesthetic agent in the subarachnoid space. Spinal anesthesia is contra-indicated in shock. Intravenous thiopentol has become a very valuable drug for induction and short operations, provided it is given slowly in a weak solution with a high concentration of oxygen in the mask. Heinwich states that the precise way in which it interferes with cellular metabolism is unknown. Overdosage of anesthetic agents is self-explanatory. Insistence by the surgeon of deep anesthesia should be carried out only at the discretion of the anesthetist.

Too heavy pre-medication or overdosage of the anesthetic agent may cause inefficient respiratory movements, thus a vicious circle occurs. Because of lack of oxygen, the medullary centers are depressed and there is a fall of blood pressure, reduced cardiac output ensues, then reduced coronary pressure results in a state of hypoxia in the myocardium, an increased carbon dioxide retention occurs, etc.

Great care and gentleness should be exercised in placing instruments or removing secretions from the nasopharynx. A reflex can be set up which can cause laryngospasm or cardiac arrest. The posterior pharynx and the carina at the bifurcation of the trachea are well known trigger areas. This must be thought of in advance in passing stomach tubes, bronchoscopes, intra-tracheal tubes, lipiodol injections of the bronchi, etc.

Definite attention and precaution must be exercised as to the position of the patient on the operating table. This has been referred to several times in the preceding pages.

In the various operative table positions there are alterations of physiology. In a great majority of operations too little thought is given to this simple fact. The cardiovascular system can be given support and protection by correct positioning.

Table rests and elevators (gall bladder and kidney) can prevent adequate chest expansion. The prone position, the lateral position, or the extreme lithotomy and extreme Trendelenburg position embarrasses respiration. An intern leaning on the chest can reduce the excursion of the chest considerably. The sitting position, while greatly interferring with the vascular system has no upsetting effect on the respiratory system.

In general no sudden change of position should occur at any time, otherwise there can be a profound and unrealistic fall of the blood pressure. This is particularly true during ether, spinal and local anesthesia. There can be a great vascular dilatation of the extremities with these drugs. If this profound fall should occur, one of the quickest ways to give the patient a transfusion is to elevate the thighs and legs to right angles, thus utilizing gravity to introduce

500 to 700 cc's. of blood into the returning venous system. Slight Trendelenburg position is some insurance against this occurrence and it is moderately good insurance against tracheal aspiration. It suffices to say that there are many uses for endotracheal anesthesia in order to insure satisfactory ventilation. In a long operation with the patient in the lateral recumbent position, it is prudent to have an intratracheal tube in place as the dependent lung is at a tremendous disadvantage.

There should be no question that the surgeon should cooperate with the anesthetist. If the anesthetist does not like the immediate condition of the patient, he should ask the surgeon to rest and in the meantime he should check all the vital signs and oxygenate the lungs well. If the surgeon proceeds blindly and does not heed the warning, it may be the difference between precipitating cardiac arrest and not. (This is particularly true in the situation, which is not a rarity, when the anesthetist finds there is a pulse, but no blood pressure recordable in the arm. Measures must then be employed which are appropriate to prevent disaster.) In a patient whose respiratory system or cardiovascular system is abnormal, either function can be brought to a halt by one of many conditions which ordinarily would not be deleterious. It may also be necessary for the surgeon to stop while the trachea is aspirated. Prolonged endotracheal aspiration is not recommended in patients with low pulmonary reserve. During cardiac surgery, runs of extra systoles and angulation of the heart may lead to a precarious state of the cardiovascular system and the alert anesthetist is usually the first to distinguish this ominous situation.

The early detection[1] of hypoxia is one of the most difficult problems in the operating room. Hypoxia is one of the most important etiological agents in the production of cardiovascular complications. Cyanosis cannot be detected by good clinical observers with good lighting conditions unless there is five grams of reduced hemoglobin. This represents only a 66 per cent oxygen saturation of the circulating hemoglobin. In the anemic person its detection is more difficult. This is referred to as occult hypoxia. The Millikan oximeter is considered good protection against hypoxia, especially the occult type. Of course, experienced anesthesiologists have other means at hand to detect hypoxia, other than being completely reliant upon the observation of cyanosis. At present there is a need for a practical instrument for measuring the CO_2 content of the expired alveolar air. The exact knowledge of the oxygen and carbon dioxide tension would enormously simplify the administration of anesthetics.

During thoracic surgery in the larger hospitals, it is now the custom to have a direct writing electrocardiograph in the operating room. This will differentiate the many serious disturbances of rhythm.

Many recorded premature beats are not recorded by the anesthetist, because they are not transmitted to the peripheral pulse. However, by far the majority of operations are done daily and will continue to be done without thought of electrocardiography.

"Monitoring" during major operations is becoming more prevalent. This means that an electronic instrument to record the electrical or sound complexes of the heart beat is attached to the patient in the operating room or recovery room. This type of recording is necessary during cardiac surgery, and its use is becoming more widespread in all fields of complicated surgery. These records still need constant careful and intelligent interpretation preferably by a cardiologist. These machines do not eliminate the need for constant attention to the many minor details which influence the physiology of the anesthetized patient. In this catastrophe the life of the patient can hinge on the early detection of cardiac stoppage. These instruments may provide one of the earliest means of its detection. Fundoscopic changes particularly those of the retinal veins, will definitely indicate cessation of the circulation within a few seconds after its occurrence.

Attention should be paid to rectal temperatures during long operations, especially in the young and old in hot weather. Elevation of temperature increases the individual's oxygen requirements. Intravenous nutrition is necessary during the course of a long operation, and also on the morning of an operation which is scheduled for the afternoon.

To reiterate, good oxygenation is one of the best means to prevent the various trigger mechanisms from taking over and precipitating this dreaded catastrophe. The best way to insure oxygenation during a great many operations is to insert an intratracheal tube.

INTRATRACHEAL INTUBATION

If the disaster unfortunately should occur with the tube in place, so much the better. One has a head start in the resuscitation procedure if the intratracheal tube is already in position.

The technique is briefly given in the following paragraphs. Skillful anesthetists state that intratracheal intubation in this emergency should not consume over thirty seconds. The patient is completely relaxed as death is imminent. The primary requirement is to have proper intratracheal tubes and a laryngoscope at hand. Various types of tubes are satisfactory. In this emergency a non-kinking endotracheal tube with inflatable cuff is preferred, because it will hold the positive pressure and also prevent aspiration into the bronchial tree. The tubes must not be too long. This is particularly true in the case of children, for the tube may extend into a bronchus and only one lung may be inflated. (A baby's trachea may be only one inch in length.)

Assuming that the patient is relaxed, there are only two remaining requirements which facilitate intratracheal intubation. They are: (1) position of the patient; (2) an understanding of the anatomy of the region of the base of the tongue in its relationship to the epiglottis.

The proper adjustment of the head and neck will result in a level straight shot from the pharynx into the trachea. The anesthetist stands behind the patient's head and places the head on a half pillow or sand bag. The back of the head is about four inches above the level of the table. The neck is then slightly flexed and the head is slightly extended. The fingers and thumb are inserted into the mouth and any excess liquid is wiped or sucked out. The teeth should be protected, but at this time this is a minor detail. Roll the lower lip outward and hold the mandible forward with the left hand.* The laryngoscope is balanced in the right hand and passed. The blade lifts the tongue upward and to the right, without trauma, until the epiglottis comes into view. Do not use the anterior teeth for a fulcrum. The lubricated tube with its concave surface away from the operator is advanced under vision through the glottis and beyond the vocal cords. Notice the vocal cords. If the cords are in spasm, the patient is not dead. Oxygen blown on them will often stimulate them to open. Connect the tube to an endotracheal adaptor and

---

*Some prefer right hand.

then to the source of oxygen. Inflate the cuff and listen for expiration of the lungs. Listen with a stethoscope to each lung. Adequate ventilation of the lungs in this procedure is a MUST. Before intubation or extubation the patient should first be well oxygenated.

In certain instances the previous technique may for some reason be impossible. Unsatisfactory insufflation of the lungs have been reported, because the endotracheal tube has been introduced into the esophagus. In other instances the proper equipment is not on hand. Under these circumstances it is proper to make use of the only life line available. This may be mouth to mouth* breathing, tracheostomy, or employment of the Kreiselman bellows. It may be necessary to lift the jaw forward, insert an oral airway, and squeeze the rubber bag. Old fashioned artificial respiration methods are practically useless and are an added hazard for the patient who is balancing on the brink of eternity.

In an extreme emergency, the oxygen saturation of the arterial blood, decreased to the point of cyanosis, may be reversed to normal, within minutes after the insertion of a large gauge oxygen[2]-carrying needle into the lumen of the trachea.

Tracheostomy should be employed more frequently, rather than postponing it to a very last re-

---

*Hold victim's nose closed.

sort. Early tracheostomy is performed with better technique and more accurate placement of the canula, if it is done before it becomes urgently necessary. The optimum level is at the third to fifth tracheal ring below the thyroid cartilage. It is important to excise a small piece of the tracheal cartilage. Such an opening permits easier insertion of the tracheostomy tube, and it prevents the edges of the trachea from sealing in case the tube should slip out.

BIBLIOGRAPHY

1. Comroe, J. H.; Botelho, S.: Unreliability of Cyanosis in the Recognition of Arterial Anoxemia. *Am. J.M. Sc., 214*:1, 1947.
2. Jacoby, J. *et al.*: Transtracheal Resuscitation *J.A.M.A., 162*:625, 1956.

X

DANGER SIGNALS OF CARDIAC ARREST

by

R. J. WHITACRE, M.D.*
Director, Department of Anesthesiology
Huron Road Hospital
Cleveland, Ohio

THE ANESTHESIOLOGIST is almost invariably in a strategic position to detect the early signs which often precede cardiac arrest during anesthesia.

The accumulated knowledge of the causes of cardiac arrest now often makes it possible to anticipate this complication. For example, we know that surgical manipulation of certain areas, such as the hilus of the lung, in the presence of inadequate anesthesia is more likely to precipitate sudden cardiac failure than when the reflexes are adequately depressed by local or general anesthesia.

There are two other causes of cardiac failure which are even more important because they occur

---

*Deceased 1956.

so much more frequently and are almost entirely under the control of the anesthesiologist. They are too high a concentration of anesthetic agent, which causes a direct depression of the heart as well as the higher centers, and a lack of oxygen. The latter cause, hypoxia, cannot be overemphasized. It is remarkable to observe how difficult it is for even experienced surgeons and anesthesiologists always to know when the tissues are adequately oxygenated. The number of patients that require cardiac resuscitation, which is so well outlined in this volume, will be greatly reduced when the causes of cardiorespiratory failure are avoided.

When acute emergencies occur, we often hear it said that the patient "suddenly went bad,"—his circulation "suddenly failed" or he "suddenly stopped breathing." As a matter of fact, what usually occurs is that it is only suddenly discovered by the anesthesiologist or surgeon that the patient is in serious difficulty. In a vast majority of cases these sudden catastrophes are preceded by definite signs which give warning of the impending failure. The prompt institution of effective therapy when the danger signals occur usually can prevent cardiac arrest.

In the past, considerable stress has been placed on the danger of a particular method of anesthesia. It is becoming increasingly well recognized that the experience and skill of the anesthesiologist are usually of much greater importance than the method of anesthesia. It is true that certain methods of anesthesia have general contraindications. Spinal anesthesia, for example, is a poor choice in the presence of shock or hemorrhage; cyclopropane is less likely to cause further depression in such cases. Pentothal ® should not be used on a patient with respiratory embarrassment. The use of too large a dose or the too rapid administration of nonvolatile drugs greatly increases the likelihood of circulatory and respiratory depression which causes tissue hypoxia and may result in cardiac arrest.

Knowing that inadequate oxygenation is a major cause of cardiac failure, it is especially important to recognize the early signs of hypoxia. The appearance of cyanosis, although important, will not always be present when the patient is hypoxic. An inadequate supply of circulating hemoglobin or pallor due to peripheral vaso-constriction, which often accompanies circulatory depression, may completely eliminate cyanosis as a dependable clinical guide. It has been demonstrated that even in normal patients, trained observers cannot always detect cyanosis until the arterial oxygen saturation is dangerously low.

Any alteration in the rate or depth of respiration should be carefully noted. A decrease in the depth or a sharp increase in the rate of respiration may interfere with adequate pulmonary ventilation and lead to hypoxia.

A progressive paralysis of the intercostal muscles due to a high level of spinal anesthesia or an increasing depth of general anesthesia should forewarn the anesthesiologist that the patient is in imminent danger. It is important to recognize that a tracheal tug or gasping type of respiration due to the unopposed action of the diaphragm may denote intercostal paralysis and impending respiratory failure.

Respiratory obstruction is one of the most common causes of cardiorespiratory failure. It is important to know that the site of obstruction may be at various levels of the respiratory tract and that appropriate means be used to correct the interference with respiratory exchange.

Accurate checking of the pulse and blood pressure every few minutes throughout the operation will provide valuable information in assessing the effectiveness of the circulation to maintain adequate tissue oxygenation. A fall in blood pressure and a marked decrease in pulse pressure that does not respond to reasonable replacement therapy, or the onset of auricular fibrillation or decompensation during anesthesia should be promptly recognized as being of serious importance. Acute hypotension of reflex origin such as may occur due to surgical manipulation usually responds to simple therapeutic measures, however, if the hypotension is uncorrected for a period of time it may gradually transcend into a situation which can cause cardiac arrest. An increase in the pulse rate to 120 or more is indicative of the

onset of surgical shock, but a slowing of the pulse to
fifty or less may indicate a decrease in the cardiac
output and be equally significant. A slowing of the
pulse rate, particularly if it precedes the stimulation
of a vagal reflex, may very well result in sudden cardiac arrest. Such patients should be adequately atro-
pinized by use of supplemental doses of atropine during anesthesia. This is becoming increasingly important due to the more frequent use of parasympatho-
mimetic drugs.

Irregularities in the pulse rate should make one
cautious toward deepening the level of anesthesia. A
decrease in skin temperature accompanied by sweat-
ing has long been known as a sign of circulatory depression.

The cerebral effects of cardiorespiratory depression are for the most part related to oxygen deficiency. Disorientation, excitement, loss of consciousness,
loss of ocular reflexes and a dilation of the pupil
should be regarded with grave importance. Muscular twitchings, particularly those that originate in
the region of the head and neck, and generalized
convulsions are very likely to be followed by circulatory failure.

At the present time, however, it is evident that
the early signs of acute cardiorespiratory failure,
though numerous, are not sharply defined. Their
recognition requires meticulous observation of the
patient at all times. No one sign can be relied upon

to the exclusion of the others. Often the earliest indications are nothing more than subtle hints or isolated signposts which, in themselves, may have no clear-cut meaning. However, if each one is carefully noted and correlated with past experience, it may indicate a trend which will alert the anesthesiologist and surgeon to institute remedial measures and thus preclude more serious complications.

XI

EQUIPMENT FOR RESUSCITATION

S PECIAL EQUIPMENT is often necessary and at times an absolute necessity for success. For all operations, regardless of the anesthesia employed certain pieces of equipment must be kept in each operating room. These instruments and equipment must be on hand and always in working order, not stored away in some obscure corner collecting cobwebs. Just because there is a Fire Department, one does not expect it to be in use twenty-four hours a day, but it must be instantly ready for all emergencies.

EQUIPMENT FOR ANESTHETIST

The anesthetist should have a special kit consisting of a laryngoscope, various intratracheal tubes, connections, lubricating jelly, and an ophthalmoscope. A rubber bag and 100 per cent oxygen should be at the head of the operating table.

RESUSCITATION KIT

An emergency sterile kit (Figure 4) should be in the operating room. It need not contain many in-

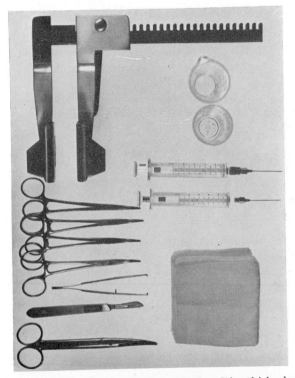

FIGURE 4. Sterile Emergency Resuscitation Kit which should
be available in every operating room. The important instruments are: Two syringes, one a metal tip, the other of glass,
a large rib spreader, a knife, and a few other instruments as
indicated. Sterile electrodes can be included in this package.

struments. It should contain a scalpel, a Finochietti retractor, two sterile medicine glasses, two 10 cubic centimeter syringes, one with a glass tip,* the other with a metal tip,* two three-inch number 22 needles, two ampules of one per cent procaine, two ampules of epinephrine,** four hemostats, surgical scissors, two electrodes, and a few sponges.

NECESSARY DRUGS

The above drugs are all that are necessary during the crisis. The surgeon should not clutter up his mind or the instrument table with others. These drugs are of proven value and there is not time to evaluate other drugs during the emergency. A tray of emergency drugs should be kept in the operating suite which can be used by consultants or assistants. This tray should contain ampules of atropine, cedelanid, ephedrine, caffeine, levartenal, mephentermine, quinidine and calcium chloride.

DEFIBRILLATOR

A shocking device or defibrillating machine is a necessity (Figure 5). In time, a hospital without a defibrillating machine will be as uncommon as a hospital without an oxygen tent is today. These ma-

---

*One for procaine and the other for epinephrine.
**Ampules are 1:1000, should be diluted with saline tenfold, it is preferred, as a large amount of solution will reach a greater portion of the myocardium through the coronary system.

chines are relatively inexpensive as compared to some operating room equipment.

In 1949, Beck and Rand[1] presented a portable fool-proof defibrillating machine at the American Medical Association meeting. After experimenting with many types and phases of currents, it was decided that one hundred and ten volts, 60 cycle, alternating current, was the best as well as the most practical, because it is used universally in this country. They found that 60 to 130 volts could be used. A large 1-1 isolation transformer is used for protection. An electrocardiograph must be disconnected at the time of the application of the shock. The amount of current used is usually one and one half to two and one half amperes. Suction cup electrodes were developed to facilitate application and rapidity of massage and they permit administering the electric shock for defibrillation at the exact moment when the heart has reached the stage of oxygenation necessary for success. This suction pulls the walls of the heart apart, so to speak, in order to make it fill better. At the same time excellent contact results.

In normal life with the chest intact the action of the heart has no suction phase. The movement of the thorax during respiration develops alternate positive and negative pressures. The pressure in the veins outside of the thorax is usually greater than in the thorax, therefore there is an aspiration or sucking effect with each inspiration which propels blood into

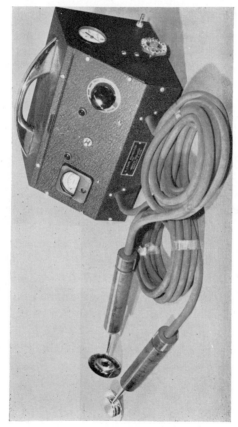

FIGURE 5. The Beck-Rand Defibrillator with suction cup electrodes. It measures eleven inches in length. Sterile pantoloons for the wires are available.

the heart.

In the present machine an outside source of vacuum is used. Most operating suites have a source of wall suction. The suction is controlled by an adjustable needle valve and registered on a gauge. About seven inches of water is normally applied.

The hazard of sparking is negligible, due to the isolation transformer. This hazard of sparking and its associated scorching effect can practically be eliminated by placing the electrodes very firmly against the myocardium. Poor contact will result in "arcing" and scorching. In the strictest sense these machines would not comply with all features of the fire code. However, the code permits the use of any equipment in order to save a life. In fact, this type of equipment does not present the hazard of ordinary x-ray equipment, which is used in the hospitals and operating rooms every day.

Experimentation has been done and is being done with the hope that a very strong current applied to the intact chest wall will prove to be the most effectual approach in the treatment of cardiac arrest. Using currents in the range above 220 volts and below 980 volts, dogs' hearts could under ideal circumstances be returned to a coordinated beat, (Fig. 6) provided that little more than 45 seconds have elapsed. About five times the amount of current is necessary to flow through the unopened chest as that is necessary when applied directly to the heart.

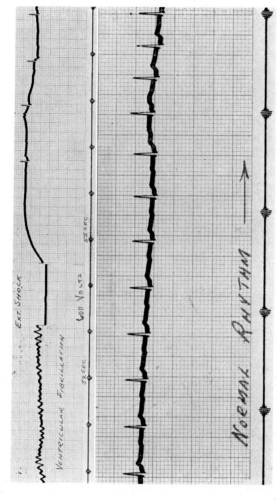

FIGURE 6. Defibrillation of a dog, following the external application of 600 volts of electricity. Chest was intact. (The E.K.G. record does not necessarily indicate as satisfactory arterial blood pressure, which is the more important.)

Zoll, in 1956, reported one successful human resuscitation from ventricular fibrillation after the application of an external defibrillation shock.

Kouwenhoven suggests: successful external defibrillation of human patients with healthy hearts and healthy lungs is entirely feasible, subject to the following conditions: (a) An external defibrillator must be immediately available. (b) Recognition of cardiac arrest must be immediate. (c) Diagnosis of ventricular fibrillation must be made. (d) Application of electric shock should take place within one minute of arrest; beyond that time successful defibrillation and recovery without prior massage becomes less and less probable.

Dow and Wiggers, in 1940, concluded that in the dog the maximum period of ventricular fibrillation which may be followed by recovery without massage is about sixty seconds.

It appears that the time limit is thus reduced about seventy-five per cent. In this vital league we are allowed only one strike. Can we afford such extravagance? We do not want to strike out before we resort to opening the chest. This approach to resuscitation, according to Beck's dictum, ignores the *EMERGENCY ACT* (Part I. the re-establishment of the oxygen system). Instead it begins with Part II (the restoration of the heart beat.) See chapter XII.

The pacemaker or heartpacer is a valuable machine to have available, particularly during the post-

resuscitative period. It cannot treat ventricular fibrillation, but applied to a patient whose heart is slow
and faltering, at times it can control and bolster the
beat and the rhythm. It is my opinion that it should
not be used during the Emergency Act. Others have
great hopes that this machine when applied to the
exterior of the body will act as a self-starter for the
arrested heart in standstill. Its main value to date
has been in the Stokes-Adams syndrome. My experience with laboratory dogs led me to believe that the
desired results will not occur after cardiac stoppage
has taken place for any ordinary length of time within the normal time limitation of three to four minutes. Its application has no effect on a dilated and
cyanotic heart. Under these circumstances when the
electrodes are applied directly to the heart, almost
without exception ventricular fibrillation occurred.
Under clinical circumstances, the greatest opportunity for success arises from first re-establishing the
oxygen system and metabolism of the myocardium.
All these various instruments can be at best nothing
but a tool, and the key to the whole subject of heart
resuscitation is the knowledge and abilities of the
attending staff.

The use of defibrillating and pacemaker machines necessitates that we as physicians have some
conception of safe current values. As has been widely
known and demonstrated, electrical currents can be
beneficial as well as extremely hazardous and harm-

ful. As paradoxical as it may seem, so-called moderately weak currents fall in the latter classification.

In the human, currents of 15 to 20 milliamperes can result in painful shock, loss of muscular control of adjacent muscles, and he cannot let go. Currents of 20 to 75 milliamperes can cause painful shock, severe muscular contractions with breathing extremely difficult. Current estimates of 75 to 200 milliamperes cause ventricular fibrillation. Current values above 200 milliamperes produce severe burns, muscular contractions, and paralysis of the respiratory center, but they prevent ventricular fibrillation. At the time the current is broken, the heart is actually defibrillated. This accounts for the amazing recoveries from short contacts with excessively high voltage. It would appear that criminals undergoing judicial electrocution forfeit their lives from the thermal effects of the current, particularly upon the brain. Within a relatively short time the body temperature will exceed 110 degrees Fahrenheit.

The use of a defibrillator upon a non-fibrillating victim appears to have little danger. The use of a pacemaker upon a fibrillating heart has no result other than to use up precious time.

MECHANICAL RESPIRATOR

In the long and difficult resuscitative procedure, a breathing machine is a definite benefit and not a luxury. A rubber bag filled with oxygen can be squeezed by hand, and the lungs can be made to inflate and deflate by this method. However, over a long period of time the Rand-Wolfe[2] respirator (Figure 7) will undoubtedly do a much better job than can be done by hand. The machine does not tire out and lose efficiency. Aeration of the lungs must meet certain requirements for success. This machine has done this.

This is an electro-mechanical respirator which is run by a spark-proof motor and switch. The breathing cycle is controlled by a cam action so designed that there is a gradual increase of bag pressure; to a peak; it is held in full inspiration for twenty-five per cent of the cycle, and then suddenly released. A very slight negative pressure develops in the expiratory phase by the sudden drop and weight of the compressing plate. The rate of positive pressure can be regulated from one to twenty-eight times per minute. The so-called rest period between each cycle should equal the length of time consumed by the breathing cycle. A short rubber breathing tube is connected from the respirator outlet to the soda lime canister of the anesthesia machine. This is a quiet running heavy duty machine which needs very little if any maintenance.

Some prefer to keep a tray of selected drugs upon a mobile cart along with oxygen tanks, face masks, rubber bag, intratracheal tubes, intravenous sets, a defibrillator and possibly a heartpacer.

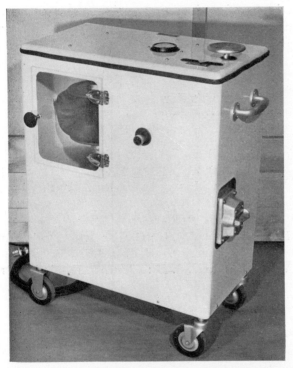

FIGURE 7. The Rand-Wolfe Mechanical Respirator which is electrically operated and is spark proof. The breathing cycle is controlled by an eccentric cam.

The anesthetist, surgeon, and hospital should always be certain that some adequate form of suction apparatus is available for possible use on the anesthetized patient in the operating room or recovery room. Intelligent use of suction will often prevent hypoxia and asphyxia in the unconcious patient.

EQUIPMENT

ANESTHETIST'S KIT
STERILE EMERGENCY KIT
EMERGENCY DRUG TRAY
BECK-RAND DEFIBRILLATING MACHINE
RAND-WOLFE RESPIRATOR
POSSIBLY A MOBILE EMERGENCY CART

BIBLIOGRAPHY

1. Beck, C. S.; Rand, J. H.: Cardiac Arrest During Anesthesia and Surgery. *J.A.M.A., 147:*1563, 1949.
2. Wolfe, K.; Rand, J. H.: Electro-mechanical Aids in Resuscitation and Anesthesia. *Ohio State M.J., 46:* 39, 1950.

XII

STEPS IN CARDIAC RESUSCITATION

IN MY OPINION the most important point in the resuscitation procedure is its SEPARATION INTO TWO DISTINCT STEPS. Beck is responsible for this basic contribution to successful resuscitation. The two components are: (1) re-establishment of the oxygen system; and (2) restoration of the heart beat. The recognition that these are two separate and distinct steps is important and has been frequently overlooked. One should not be confused with the other. The re-establishment of the oxygen system is the emergency act. Knowledge of each of these steps is just as important as knowledge of the other. The importance of each simple step cannot be overemphasized, as failure in one may often account for failure to save a life. This concept focuses attention on the oxygen system, not on the heart beat, in which we naturally tend to show the greater interest. With a thorough understanding of this distinction, the problem of resuscitation becomes simple, provided one can place and keep first things first and can exert the necessary perseverance.

It is also important to know the THINGS TO DO and the THINGS NOT TO DO during those critical moments when a life is hanging in the balance. Too often in the past, temporizing time-consuming measures have been carried out which are things not to do. This has been particularly true of those surgeons in the specialty groups. Because they are not familiar with abdominal or thoracic surgery they are reluctant to slit open the chest. They would employ all measures short of this. In the meantime the oxygen deficiency of the brain has resulted in permanent damage.

If the proper procedure is carried out we would like to believe that any normal heart that has stopped can be made to beat again. This is not a ridiculous or boastful statement, for it refers to the occasional patient whose heart for all intents and purposes is normal, but rather suddenly and unexpectedly ceases to beat during an anesthetic induction or during an operation. The foregoing statement has been carefully worded. It assumes, first, that there is no inherent cardiac disease, second, that arrest has occurred in the operating room, and third, that all the correct and necessary steps have been carried out within the accepted time limitation.

In the past, instances of successful and complete cardiac resuscitation have been too few and too far between. There are three major reasons for this failure: (1) lack of a plan of attack; (2) failure to act within the time limitation; and (3) severe inherent cardiac disease. The principal factor in the first reason for failure is a lack of understanding of the real problem by the persons involved. The second reason revolves around the surgeon's inhibitions about opening the chest. He feels that he must make sure the patient is at least 200 per cent dead, otherwise he may be criticized by his colleagues. The last reason is self-explanatory.

As has been previously stated and will be mentioned over and over again, the re-establishment of the oxygen system is the emergency act. Once this system is established, the crisis is over because the heart beat can be restored without special reference to time. In fact, another surgeon might be summoned from some distance to restore the heart beat or to bring a defibrillating machine. (This was done in Chicago in 1951. The machine was brought across town by police escort and a student nurse was successfully restored to life.)

A definite step by step plan must be put into effect. The surgeon must be so geared to this that in the confusion he can perform the proper steps reflexly and conquer his inertia. Most failures are attributed to the limitation of time. This time limitation of three to five minutes must be overcome, otherwise the patient's brain is irreversibly damaged, although the heart beat and circulation is returned to normal.

Once cardiac arrest occurs, it is important to know what should be done as well as what should not be done. There is no time to improvise. The surgeon is on the spot. He must instinctively be able to do the right thing. Dynamic consequences result from making a wrong step or from indecision. Time must not be taken to demonstrate to everyone in the operating room that the patient is absolutely and unquestionably dead. If there is no pulse in the large arteries, no blood pressure, no respirations, and pupillary dilatation, the patient for all intents and purposes is dead.

Kevorkian in 1956 has recalled to the attention of those interested in resuscitation, the changes in the retinal vessels which are indicative of impending and of actual death. These changes can act as an important clinical guide to differentiate profound shock from cardiac arrest and can be of importance in estimating the elapsed time after death. Beading or segmentation of veins of the retina almost invariably is observed within several seconds after cardiac output ceases. This beading with movement can continue up to ten to twenty minutes. No known clinical aid can determine so quickly whether or not the circulation has stopped.

Bouchut, in 1864, one year after the invention of the ophthalmoscope, reported on some new signs of death furnished by this instrument. He reported that with "granular movement" there is cardiac standstill, but it does not necessarily mean death, and recovery is possible. In 1906, Albrand-Sachsenberg placed emphasis on the use of these fundscopic signs in determining resuscitability or the remote possibility of premature interrment.

In 1939, the author stood at the head of a patient who had had a massive hemothrax with resultant shift of the mediastinum. Another physician was aspirating the blood from the chest. The pupils abruptly became widely dilated. Immediately, I viewed the fundi with an ophthalmoscope. I was amazed when the veins became segmented and noticed the movement or flow of these segments. This commenced as I observed the eye grounds.

My own physiological interpretation at the time was that death at that moment had supervened, and the movement was dependent upon the resiliency of the peripheral circulatory system. The ancients always found the aorta empty as its muscular had "milked" the blood along. The term aorta referred to an air tube. It was not until Harvey's discovery in 1628 that it was learned that the aorta did not transport air. In the meantime I have overlooked this important clinical sign as an indication of cessation of the circulation.

THINGS NOT TO DO

The operator must not miss an opportunity for success by using precious moments to carry out incorrect actions. The inclinations of those who do not comprehend the problem might lead them to make one of the following mistakes.

(1) Do not attempt to administer artificial respiration by compression of the thoracic cage.

(2) Do not listen for faint heart sounds. In the confusion and with wishful hearing one is apt to hear his own heart beat. If there is no palpable pulse in the large arteries and no measurable blood pressure and if respiration has ceased, the surgeon can be

certain that any slight movement of the heart is of no consequence.

(3) Do not change the blood pressure cuff to the other arm.

(4) Do not wait for an electrocardiogram. Furthermore, electrical impulses may be recorded four to six minutes after visible cessation of the heart beat (Figure 8).

(5) Do not inject epinephrine through the chest wall into the heart.

(6) Do not give a blood transfusion.

(7) Do not give an arterial blood transfusion.

(8) Do not dilate the rectal sphincter.

(9) Do not make an abdominal incision in order to attempt subdiaphragmatic cardiac massage.

(10) Do not try intramuscular or intravenous medication.

(11) Do not strike the chest repeatedly.

PART I. Re-establishment of the Oxygen

System (The Emergency Act)

In the re-establishment of the oxygen system, oxygen must be delivered into the lungs and blood, and the oxygenated blood must be circulated effectively. The anesthetist must be on his toes and alert. The first thing he must do is to insert a properly fit-

---

A "Pace Maker" has no place in Part I, but it may have a place at the end of Part II in assisting the heart beat.

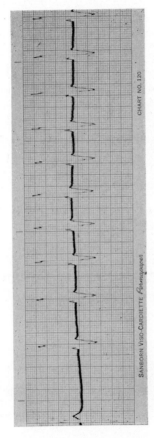

FIGURE 8. Electrocardiogram taken after five minutes of cardiac standstill with no visible contraction of the heart.

ting tube into the trachea and then inflate and deflate the lungs adequately by compression of a rubber bag filled with 100 per cent oxygen. This is the foundation of success. If a tube is already in place before cardiac failure occurs, so much the better. However this maneuver should not occupy more than 30 seconds of time, as the patient is completely relaxed. Any hesitation in carrying this out is the first step toward disaster. This responsibility belongs to the anesthetist as the surgeon at this point has too many other vital obligations. Knowing that oxygen is being delivered to the patient, the surgeon remembers additional things which should NOT be done in this emergency.

Additional Things Not To Do

1. Do not Take Time for Asepsis.

2. Do not Shave the Chest.

3. Do not Drape the Chest.

4. Do not Count the Interspaces before Making Incision.

It is obvious that not a second can be wasted. Even a small amount of air made available in the lungs, may accomplish what pure oxygen and adequate pulmonary ventilation may fail to do fifteen to thirty seconds later. The moment that the anesthetist can adequately aerate the lungs, the surgeon boldly proceeds to incise* the chest in order to

---

*A small incision can be made first. If there is no active bleeding, there is no circulation.

squeeze the heart which will in turn circulate the oxygenladen blood. In the meantime someone in the operating room should be designated to call out the* minutes. Time should not be spent on asepsis. Matters such as shaving, cleansing the skin, draping the patient and putting on sterile gloves are subordinate and hardly need comment. The surgeon does not count the interspaces, but estimates the position of the fourth or fifth left interspace and makes a quick and deliberate intercostal incision from the sternum to the underlying sheet (Figure 9). There is no bleeding because there is no blood pressure. Later the internal mammary artery may have to be secured; this is to be hoped for. It is preferred to have the left arm outstretched on a board or abducted.

It is well to realize that the heart may be quite dilated and somewhat larger than expected. At times it has been nicked with the scalpel as the bold incision is made. This is of no consequence, as later it can easily be sutured. The phrenic nerve lies well posteriorly, while the vagus nerves are in close association with the esophagus at this level.

The right hand is now thrust into the chest cavity pushing the lung posteriorly and is guided behind the heart and the intact pericardium. An assistant may hold the ribs apart. The heart is lifted upward

---

*Later it may be hard to recapture the time sequence of events.

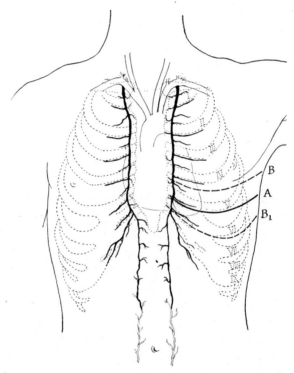

FIGURE 9. Thorax showing incision in fifth left I. C. S. (A) alternate incisions (B and B_1). Position of internal Mammary Artery is indicated.

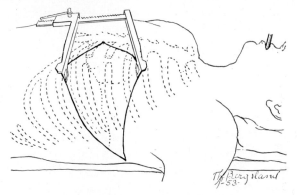

FIGURE 9. (Continued).

and compressed against the sternum and massage commenced.* The crisis is now over, the oxygen system is functioning. The patient is now protected. The brain can be kept alive and the surgeon can begin to relax and to think. A call for a consultant can be placed. The anesthetist can adjust the table to a 10 degree Trendelenburg position. By this time the operator's wrist may be virtually strangulated between the ribs, so he pauses long enough to cut the costochondral arches of the two adjacent ribs, thus permitting more room. Immediately, additional manual massage is undertaken, remembering that any pause results at once in an ineffectual circul-

---

*For technique see page 132.

ation. A short time later a large self-retaining retractor* is introduced, and the pericardium can be opened longitudinally from base to apex. Quickly the heart is grasped in the hand and massage again instituted. By this time the anesthetist should see a noticeable change in the patient's color. Now it is desirable to have an assistant take over in a sterile gown and gloves. The surgeon may find that his forearm is extremely tired. He rests by cleansing the field and putting on sterile gloves and gown. If the heart beat has not been restored at this stage, the operator returns to manual massage of the heart. Several teams should be available if necessary, as it is hard and strenuous work. A blood pressure adequate to maintain life can be sustained in this fashion for as long as eight hours, as it was in a patient who is now a practicing lawyer in New York City.**

Thus the first and most important part of the emergency procedure has been inaugurated. The oxygen system has been re-established. Oxygen is getting into the lungs and being circulated to the vital organs by an effective blood pressure. The patient can be kept alive indefinitely. The next step in the resuscitation procedure must now be undertaken, that is, to restore the normal heart beat. This can be done minutes or hours later.

---

*Do not compress the heart against the blade of the retractor.

**M. N. Foote: Personal communication to the author in 1950.

Up to this juncture, it is not known whether the heart is in standstill or in ventricular fibrillation. Since the procedure for resuscitation is somewhat different in the two conditions, the surgeon now stops massage momentarily and observes the ventricles. If there are no fibrillary movements, he can assume that the heart is in a state of asystole or standstill.

PART II. Restoration of the Heart Beat

CARDIAC STANDSTILL

A. Method of Restoring Heart Beat in Cardiac Asystole. The heart in asystole may start beating after hand massage alone. The less time that has elapsed since failure of the circulation, the more readily it can be made to beat again. The heart may without difficulty start beating after massage through the intact pericardium and may run away just as winding a watch. At times the ease with which the heart beat can be restored is unbelievable. The normal heart will beat if given the chance. If the heart should not resume its rhythmic beat after adequate massage has been carried out for several minutes, 3 to 5 cc's. of one to ten thousand (1:10,000) epinephrine solution is injected into the chamber of the right ventricle and massage is continued. It is best to use a long, number 22 needle and insert it diagonally through the myocardium and withdraw on the plunger so as to be sure it is in the lumen or chamber. Diagonally inserting the needle results in a self-seal. The needle should not injure a coronary vessel. The massage perfuses the epinephrine through the heart and then to the aorta, coronary arteries, and thus into the myocardium.

Preference of the site for the injection of drugs varies. Most authors state that ventricular injections are prone to cause ventricular fibrillation if made into a solitary site in the myocardium, because it acts as a hyper-irritable focus. The right ventricle is preferred because it does not bleed as easily as the auricle; it is more accessible and has fewer coronary vessels on its presenting surface than the left ventricle. Its wall is less thick than the left ventricle, and it does not have the large papillary muscles of the left chamber. However, the matter of the injection site is of minor importance in this formidable emergency.

In many instances the heart will then begin to beat if all conditions are favorable. If it fails to do so, the surgeon should check the excursion of the lungs and observe the color of the myocardium. The color of the myocardium is a very valuable sign as it indicates the effectiveness of the restoration of the oxygen system. Good oxygenation of the lungs and adequate blood flow to the myocardium are essential in any attempt to revive the heart.

If after three to five minutes of adequate massage there is still no heart beat, epinephrine can be injected for a second and third time and warm saline can be poured on the surface of the heart. If success has not been achieved, an electrocardiogram should be made to make certain that the heart is not in imperceptible ventricular fibrillation. If the heart is not in fibrillation and fails to produce coordinated beats, the reason may be faulty aeration of the lungs, faulty massage of the heart, peripheral circulatory failure, or intrinsic cardiac disease. The importance of movement of the lungs is emphasized. When cardiac resuscitation is difficult and the procedure prolonged, a mechanical respirator is of great assistance and may mean the difference between success and failure. I prefer the Rand-Wolfe respirator (Figure 7) because it guarantees the proper transport of oxygen at a regular rate and during a long procedure does not tire out and lose its efficiency. Inadequate oxygenation of the blood and inadequate elimination of carbon dioxide are the common causes of failure to restore the heart beat. Beck states that repeated injections of large doses of epinephrine cause the myocardium to become refractory to this drug. When such a stage is reached, ampules of calcium chloride may be substituted.

VENTRICULAR FIBRILLATION

B. Method of Restoring Beat in Ventricular Fibrillation. During ventricular fibrillation the heart muscle is in a state of convulsion. A convulsion is a purposeless movement of muscle bundles. There is such incoordination of the muscle fibers that the blood pressure is not maintained. Within two or three seconds after its onset, the blood pressure ab‧ruptly falls to zero (Figure 1) .

In general, the method of defibrillation requires that steps be taken to abolish fibrillation before the coordinated beat can be restored, but massage (Figure 10) is still the most important component since it overcomes the dilatation and anoxia of the heart. Cardiac massage is carried out long enough to insure good color and tone of the heart muscle. An electric shock is usually required at this juncture. It is applied by placing a good sized electrode on each side (ventricle) of the heart** so that as much muscle mass as possible lies between them. The electrodes are then squeezed together to displace the blood and make good contact. Care must be taken to make sure the operator is protected by insulation, as it is within the realm of possibilities to have two candidates for defibrillation instead of one. The handles of the electrodes should be heavily insulated and the surgeon should always wear intact gloves after having removed any ring. A shock is then applied for one long* second, as in saying "one thousand." During the second that the current flows through the heart,

*Some defibrillators have an automatic timer.
**Moisten with warm saline solution.

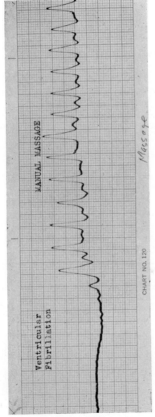

FIGURE 10. Effective blood pressure developed while heart is fibrillating. Cessation of massage results in an immediate fall to zero with all its dynamic consequences.

all the muscle fibers and bundles are again coordinated, they are in a state of contraction. When the current is broken they all relax together, and it is hoped that the A-V node will send down the stimulus which will result in a coordinated beat (Figure 11). Failure means a resumption of fibrillation.

If a coordinated beat results, epinephrine and massage are used in the manner already described in the technique for standstill. Often it remains motionless for several seconds, then suddenly there is a forceful beat almost like a large gulp. At other times it will resume its coordinated rhythm with weak ineffectual beats. This latter type must be helped along by manual massage and at the same time a close watch is kept to make sure the heart does not slip back into fibrillation. This is referred to as assisted cardiac massage.

If fibrillation continues or recurs, massage is continued and the shock procedure repeated. If this is done several times without success an injection of 3-5 cc's of one per cent procaine is injected into the chamber of the right ventricle. Cold saline can be poured upon the surface of the heart. The use of procaine at this point in the difficult case often means the difference between success and failure. If fibrillation still persists and muscular tone is poor, massage of the heart is continued and a small dose of epinephrine is used. To administer epinephrine in the face of fibrillation is contrary to physiological

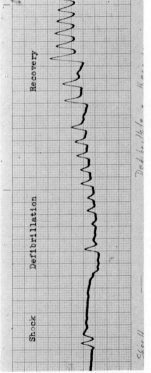

FIGURE 11. The heart is brought out of fibrillation. There is progressive rise of blood pressure as the coordinated beat is resumed.

principles, nevertheless Beck's experience, as well as mine, indicates that it can be effective. It can restore tone and supply the stimulus that initiates the beat after the next shock. If the heart beat is not restored after many attempts, the surgeon must consider the following possibilities: (1) anoxia of the heart muscle; (2) retention of carbon dioxide; (3) procaine effect; (4) the epinephrine effect; and (5) intrinsic cardiac disease.

The first two possibilities may indicate poor massage technique, poor ventilation of the lungs, or insufficient blood volume.

In certain instances the heart beat appears somewhat satisfactory on inspection, yet an ineffectual blood pressure is attained. This could be due to peripheral vascular collapse, and one of the most direct ways of combating this is to give an intra-arterial transfusion into the aorta.

In difficult cases, circulation of the blood and ease of application of the electrical shock can be improved by the use of the Beck-Rand suction cup electrodes, particularly when the heart has lost its muscular tone and there is collapse of the peripheral vascular tree. The suction helps fill the chambers of the hydrodynamic pump, and the heart can be squeezed as many as 120 beats per minute without having one's forearm feel as if it were to fall off. Although the effective blood pressure is not appreciably greater than that produced by manual massage, the volume of blood circulated is greater, and if the volume is greater, the amount of oxygen circulated is also greater.

The *secret* to success in these instances is to have the body and heart muscle in a good state of oxygenation (Figure 12). Other workers in this field logically suggest that during prolonged massage, the descending thoracic aorta be clamped off so that the blood manually ejected from the heart is directed to the brain and coronary arteries. In the prolonged procedure, it is questionable whether or not this is the proper step to carry out, as our laboratory group feel that the adrenal glands are second only to the brain in vulnerability to lack of oxygen. Newer concepts of the function of the liver indicate that the anoxic liver in shock elaborates a vaso-depressor substance, or it fails to secrete a sustaining factor. *In the ladder of descendency,* the kidneys are probably fourth in vulnerability.

If this specific procedure seems feasible at this juncture of the resuscitation, the aorta can be pinched, not clamped, for alternate periods of thirty seconds or so. If the descending aorta is occluded longer, carbon dioxide is accumulated in the peripheral vascular tree with resultant vaso-dilation. Upon release of the aorta a greater degree of hypotension is encountered as a larger reservoir is created.

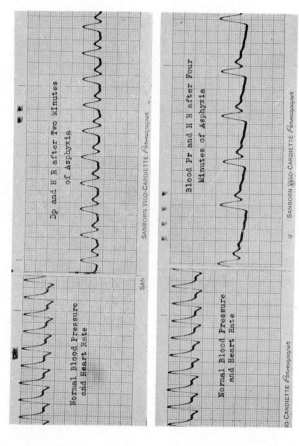

FIGURE 12. Development of bradycardia and hypotension from anoxia.

PART I. THE EMERGENCY ACT
STEP BY STEP PROGRAM OF ACTION
FOR RE-ESTABLISHMENT OF THE
OXYGEN SYSTEM

ANESTHETIST

Notify surgeon of impending death
Note pupils and fundi
Have surgeon check pulse in large arteries
Note time
Insert intratracheal tube
Expand lungs by squeezing bag of oxygen
Direct attendant to extend left arm (if possible)
Lower head of table slightly

SURGEON

Boldly make long incision in left fifth intercostal
space
Insert hand and squeeze heart against sternum
Susbsequently pause to cut costochondral arches
Resume massage for one to two minutes
Insert Finochietti rib retractor
Resume massage
Open pericardium longitudinally
Grasp heart with one or both hands and mas-
sage
Pause momentraily, observe heart
Standstill?   Ventricular Fibrillation?

PART II

STEP BY STEP PROGRAM FOR RESTORATION OF HEART BEAT

STANDSTILL

Continue massage

If not successful, inject three to five c.c.'s of 1:10,000 epinephrine into right ventricle

Quickly resume massage

Repeat injections if necessary

FIBRILLATION

Continue massage until myocardium is pink

Quickly and accurately apply electrodes

Deliver countershock from defibrillation machine

If unsuccessful, continue massage

After a few shocks, 1 per cent procaine (three to four c.c.'s) is injected into right ventricle

Resume massage

Apply shock

If successful, carry out program for standstill

CLOSURE

Do not be in a hurry to close chest

Secure internal mammary artery

Intravenous atropine 1/150 grain ⎫

1 AMP (4 c.c.) cedilanid   ⎬ I. V.

Intravenous 20% glucose   ⎭

XIII

METHODS OF CARDIAC
MASSAGE

I T IS DIFFICULT to tell someone how to massage a
heart so that it will resume its function as a satisfactory hydrodynamic pump. Actual experience is
the only teacher. One must get the feel of the blood
surging out of the heart beneath the fingers. Once
this feel or know-how is developed one can be quite
certain that one is producing an effective circulation.

Purposeless squeezing of the heart is like paw-
ing the air; nothing happens as far as satisfactory
blood pressure is concerned. The student becomes
aware of this as he massages the heart for the first
time. The blood pressure is recorded by an electromanometer, and he is able to visualize the pressure
he is producing. Much to his surprise and chagrin,
in the beginning it will read 20-25 mm. of mercury.
After a short time with instruction and more care in
emptying the right ventricle, he finds he is able to
sustain a blood pressure of 75-100 mm.

There are several ways to massage the arrested
heart; however they all depend upon the basic prin-
ciple—it is necessary to empty both ventricles.

MASSAGE WITH INTACT PERICARDIUM

Massage can be carried out through the intact pericardium with the chest open. It is necessary to do this when the chest is first opened in order to restore the oxygen system at the earliest moment. The heart is lifted up and compressed flatly against the inferior surface of the sternum. At this stage the rib retractor has usually not been placed (Figure 13). If so, care must be exercised not to compress the ventricle against the blade of the retractor. However, it is doubtful with this method, that a satisfactory blood pressure can be developed which will keep the brain alive for an indefinite period. Other methods are more fruitful.

SUBDIAPHRAGMATIC APPROACH

In the first successful cases, the subdiaphragmatic approach was used. Today, it is not recommended, because in that method a satisfactory blood pressure cannot be maintained, and if the heart is in a state of ventricular fibrillation the operator will be unaware of it. There are reports of successful subdiaphragmatic massage, but we do not read of the many failures. If the surgeon has an upper abdominal incision open, it is permissible to make an attempt to massage the heart through the diaphragm. If the heart fails to beat, more than ten seconds should not be spent on this maneuver. Those hearts which resume their normal beat probably do so from the mechanical stimu-

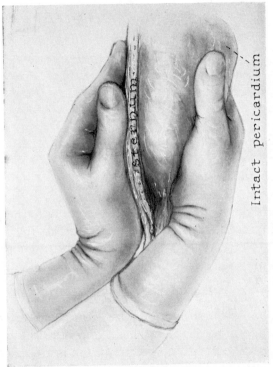

FIGURE 13. Cardiac Massage (Human Heart).

lation of "poking" through the diaphragm, as satisfactory manual massage is impossible.

TRANSDIAPHRAGMATIC APPROACH

The transdiaphragmatic approach from within
the abdominal cavity is accomplished by retracting
the left lobe of the liver to one side and incising the
leaf of the diaphragm just behind the sternum. This
allows somewhat better manual massage than the
preceding maneuver.

TRANSTHORACIC APPROACH

It is strongly recommended that the chest be
opened in the resuscitation procedure. It will contribute greatly to the operator's chance of success.
A generous intercostal incision is necessary. It should
extend from the left border of the sternum to the underlying sheet. It is good surgical practice today to
make a thoracotomy, if there is any reasonable doubt
concerning the adequacy of the heart action.

MASSAGE WITH ONE HAND

The best method for massaging the heart depends upon the size of the heart and the size of the
surgeon's hands. After exposure of the heart, the operator, on the left side of the table, places his right
hand around the heart with the wrist in slight ulnar
deviation and dorsi-flexion. The fingers are placed
along the border of the left ventricle and the thumb

and thenar eminence around the lateral border of the
right ventricle (Figure 14). The heart is then delib-
erately, but gently, squeezed in a rhythmic fashion.
An important feature is—*relaxation of the hand
must be an active process.* It is done actively, quickly, and precisely by using the extensor muscles of the
hand and forearm. If the hand is slowly relaxed and
allowed to surround the heart in the diastolic phase,
the weight and pressure of the hand alone will interfere with cardiac filling. There is a knack and feel
which one soon learns from actual experience. The
blood can be felt to surge and pulsate out of the
chambers beneath one's fingers. Care must be exercised to insure that the right ventricle is being
emptied. Failure to do so is the usual mistake of the
novice. It is natural to concentrate upon the left
ventricle, as it is intimately concerned with the
systemic blood pressure. However, in order for the
left ventricle to fill, the right ventricle must be emptied of blood and subsequently fill the left ventricle.

To repeat, manual massage is deliberate and
purposeful, but the myocardium must not be
squeezed to the point of injury to insure that every
drop of blood has been ejected from its chambers,
for this conception is unphysiological. Normally the
chambers of the ventricles are never entirely obliter-
ated; there always remains a small cylindrical space.
In this maneuver it is important to remember that
the onset of normal ventricular contraction is sud-

den, so this may be duplicated manually. There is a quick rise of pressure in the chambers that balloons out and presses the flaps of the mitral and tricuspid valves together. If the manual massage is carried on slowly and lazily, these valves become incompetent. In other words, this maneuver is not like wringing out a dish rag!

Attention must be paid to make sure one does not angulate the heart, for if this is done the great vessels at its base will be constricted. The fingers and hand should not surround the thin auricles. It is possible to injure the auricles and sometimes the ventricles by too vigorous manipulation. Do not dig the tips of the fingers into the myocardium. If the finger punctures the myocardium, it should be quickly sutured. Such a puncture can occur in the area of an infarct (see Case History VII). The amount of trauma the myocardium will withstand without causing any serious or permanent injury is remarkable.

MASSAGE WITH BOTH HANDS

In some instances, especially with the larger hearts, the fingers of the left hand can be placed in front of the heart, and the palm and fingers of the right hand behind the heart, and the left hand kept more or less stationary (Figure 14). Massage is carried out by moving the right hand toward the left one. The walls of the ventricles should always be compressed against the inter-ventricular septum.

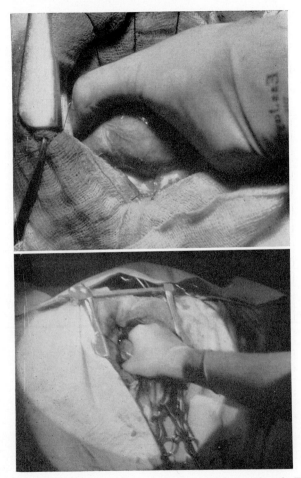

FIGURE 14. Cardiac massage carried on with one hand. The fingers of the right hand surround the left ventricle and the thumb lies across the right ventricle. The anterior descending coronary artery delineates the right and left chambers.

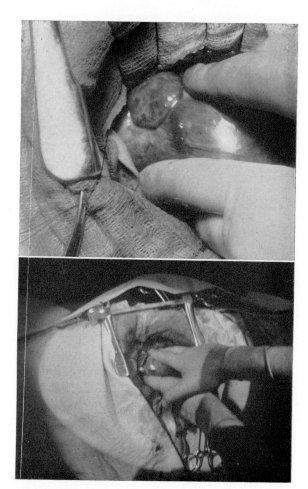

FIGURE 14. (Continued).
Upper—illustrates "assisted massage," (page 139).
Each hand placed flatly over each ventricle. The walls are
then compressed toward the interventricular septum.

The fingers should not include the auricle. In small children two fingers on each side of the heart are used. (In the newborn, mouth to mouth breathing and squeezing the heart between the thumb and index finger will establish the oxygen system.)

ASSISTED MASSAGE

When the heart is beating feebly it is a good plan to assist its emptying by manually compressing it every second or third beat to facilitate the emptying of its chambers. This will often help it through a precarious situation when one is not sure whether or not it will stop or continue to beat. The best way to do this is to place two fingers of each hand on either side of the heart. In this way the operator can look down between his hands and observe the character of the beat. With one hand covering the heart, this hand must be withdrawn from the chest in order to observe the beat, which is a distinct disadvantage.

RATE OF MASSAGE

The rate of massage depends upon the filling of the heart. If the rate is too fast, one quickly notices that the heart is not filling properly, and insufficient systemic blood pressure results. It is physically difficult to carry out manual massage for any length of time at a rate of over sixty to seventy squeezes per minute.

SUCTION CUP MASSAGE

In 1949, Beck and Rand experimented with methods of mechanical massage of the arrested heart. The devices could not do better than could be done by manual massage. Both methods squeezed the heart and emptied it. Neither method influenced diastolic filling. Suction cup electrodes (Figure 5) were devised which when placed on each ventricle gently pulled its walls apart as in a bellows action. This helped fill the arrested heart with blood. The pulse waves could readily be increased up to one hundred twenty per minute. Although the blood pressure peak was not higher, more volume of blood could be moved each minute. Therefore more oxygenated blood could be circulated. The electric countershock could readily be applied without the prolonged pause for applying electrodes. The gentle suction held the metal electrodes on the slippery organ, thus making better contact. It is observed that the inexperienced operator can sustain a better blood pressure with use of the suction cups.

In using this special instrument, the electrode in the left hand is held almost stationary, while the right one undergoes the major excursion. This procedure is definitely less tiring than manual massage. These electrodes are made in various sizes, the average being 6.5 cm. in diameter. They are not a necessity but they are worthwhile pieces of operating room equipment.

XIV

CLOSURE OF THE CHEST

THE SURGEON should not be in a hurry to close the chest as soon as the heart starts to beat. It is a natural and human reaction, once the heart beat has been restored, to want to run away from the ordeal. There can not be a let down of events. The heart beat should be carefully observed for a period of time; this time depends upon the individual surgeon's judgment. It is desirable to give at least 1/100th or 1/150th grain of atropine intravenously at this time. Intravenous administration of fluids or a transfusion may be judiciously started.

If the surgeon is satisfied with the heart action and blood pressure, the pericardium can be closed. It is closed loosely with interrupted sutures. They should be spaced far enough apart to permit fluid to drain into the pleural cavity, yet close enough to prevent the heart from herniating through the peri-cardial opening. It is not an absolute necessity to close the pericardium, but it is advisable. The excess fluid which accumulates in the pleural sinus may be aspirated several days later.

Herniations of the heart through a pericardial

fenestra have been described. The heart protrudes through the opening until the thin-walled auricles are compressed by the ring of pericardial tissue. This results in compression of the heart with poor, if any, filling of its chambers and an increased venous pressure.

Before closing the chest wall incision, be positive that the internal mammary artery is ligated. The incision is closed by placing a row of pericostal absorbable sutures which include the adjacent ribs. The costal cartilages are sutured. Then a Bailey rib approximator may be used to hold the ribs in their proper position. Rake retractors or Lambotte bone-holding forceps may be used in place of the Bailey clamp. In small children the assistant can hold the adjacent ribs in place with his fingers. The pericostal sutures are now tied. The remainder of the chest wall is closed in layers. The chest is tightly closed and before the last suture is tied, a rubber catheter removes the entrapped air in the pleural cavity. The lungs are fully inflated, and at this moment the catheter is removed and the last suture is tied. A catheter may be brought out through the thoracic wall which drains the pleural space for forty-eight to seventy-two hours. It is necessary to have a water seal type of drainage in this instance. An elastic type of adhesive holds the dressing in place.

Upon completion of the closure of the chest, the patient may be carefully transferred to his bed in the operating room if his condition warrants it. The patient should NOT be taken directly to the ward. He is kept either in the operating room or adjoining recovery room for several hours. This room should not be hot. A temperature of 68°-70° F is preferred. Hot water bottles to the extremities are not recommended. Some prefer ice bags. The intratracheal tube should be left in place as it may be necessary to keep the patient on mechanical respiration for some time. A Drinker respirator may at times be useful, as well as an oxygen tent. Sedation may be necessary to relieve restlessness.

Intravenous fluids or transfusions should be given judiciously and not routinely. Human serum albumin may be administered intravenously to combat cerebral edema if arrest has bordered on the normal time limitation. The value of vasopressor drugs is not clear except in the incipient or acute phase of shock. We prefer levarterenol bitartrate in a constant drip. There is also a place for adrenal cortex extracts in those cases in which there is a gradual and steady decline of blood pressure. One half the digitalizing* dose of Cedilanid is recommended before complete closure of the chest.

If the heart beat has been successfully restored, the question of postponement of the operation en-

---

*Usually 1 ampoule. (4cc) ; Beck has found that all his cardiac cases and all major surgical patients over fifty years of age, do much better if pre-operative digitalization is carried out.

ters the picture. In the middle of a complicated operation there may be no choice other than to finish the operation in the safest and quickest method. Continuing an elective operation rests upon the judgment of the surgeon, but in the majority of instances it is prudent and like removing a lode stone, to postpone or discontinue the operation. In the great majority of instances this unheralded catastrophe will not occur again upon another day.

XV

POST-OPERATIVE
MANAGEMENT

IT IS EXTREMELY important to be absolutely certain
of an adequate airway at all times during the immediate post-operative period. The intratracheal
tube should not be removed until it is ascertained
the patient will take over breathing on his own. The
respiratory function can be mechanically controlled
for several hours by this method. A Drinker respirator may be useful.

The blood pressure, pulse, and respiratory rate
should be recorded every five minutes for the first
few hours. Sometimes the blood pressure gradually
ebbs away in spite of the use of intravenous fluids
and vasopressors. Mephentermine (10-25 mgs. intravenously) * is effectual without appreciably accelerating the heart rate. Levarterenol (4cc's. to 1000cc's.
of fluid) combats hypotension without accelerating
the heart. Neosnephrin in the amount of 1 cc. of 1
per cent solution to 500cc's. of fluid is a very satisfactory drug. The new adrenal cortex extracts may be
particularly efficacious as the adrenals may have suf-

*Or by intravenous drip 40 mgs. to 200 cc's of fluid.

fered from the deprivation of oxygen. From extensive animal and human studies it appears that adrenal cortical hormones restore sensitivity to the vascular bed to vasopressors. In periods of acute stress the body need for hydrocortisone increases; if the adrenals fail to meet this need, shock may develop and the patient becomes increasingly unresponsive to vasoconstrictors. One such hormone which may be given is hydrocortisone sodium succinate, given intravenously in 100 milligram amounts every three hours.

Fluids must be given judiciously, and one must depend a great deal on the patient's response to the treatment. Blood is recognized as the fluid without a rival for its excellence in the treatment of existent circulatory disturbances, especially for replacement of blood volume. If blood is not immediately available, plasma will temporarily suffice for replacement of volume. During this period the circulatory system will not tolerate overloading. At times compression bandages are used to prevent blood from pooling in the extremities and abdomen.

Acute cerebral edema is usually the cause of death in those individuals whose circulatory systems have been restored to normalcy. This may occur several hours or several days later. In those cases in which there is a question as to whether the period of cerebral anoxia was within three minutes, it is advised that twenty-five per cent human serum albumin be administered intravenously in one hundred cubic centimeter amounts every four hours or as often as it appears necessary. The usual methods to promote dehydration are also carried out. Clinicians and investigators are not entirely in accord with the indications for administering corticotropin or hydrocortisone to allay cerebral edema. The rationale is that unless there has been complete destruction of brain tissue, corticotropin may suppress inflammation, thereby reducing the swelling and pressure, and lead to better circulation in the brain.

Seldon[1] made the following interesting and important observation regarding damage to the brain resulting from a period of cerebral anoxia. "It is suggested that a considerable portion of the permanent damage reported in these unfortunate cases may be the result not of the initial insult, but rather a period of untreated cerebral edema subsequent to the initial insult." Intravenous barbitrates are usually necessary to control convulsions.

The patient should be kept in flat or slight Trendelenburg position until reaction is complete. The unoperated side should always be up and free.

An oxygen tent may serve to supply additional oxygen and to act as a cooling medium. Other cooling procedures—applying ice bags and giving alcohol rubs are employed. The total fluid intake and output are recorded each twenty-four-hour period. Rou-

tine and special laboratory procedures will be required as various problems present themselves. The
nurse should be alert for signs of renal failure which
indicate a lower nephron syndrome.

The room should be cool and only light gar-
ments should be used. The patient's temperature
should be taken every hour for the first eight hours.
A rapid rise in temperature usually indicates cerebral injury.

After six years,[2] the place of hypothermia in the
treatment of cerebral anoxia and myocardial anoxia
has not been satisfactorily evaluated. In 1951 it was
suggested by us to a surgeon for intracardiac surgery.
Eleven months later on August 28, 1952, he carried
out the first intracardiac surgery in a human under
hypothermic conditions.

Cardiac disturbances must usually be diagnosed
with the aid of a consultant and electro-cardiograph.
This is especially true in the diagnosis of certain disorders of rhythm. The following drugs have been
found helpful. They should be kept in the operating
room and recovery room on a special tray in ampule
form. These may be used, preferably, by the consultant. (The surgeon should not clutter up his operating table or brain with other drugs than procaine
and epinephrine as he has too many other vital
obligations. These are the two drugs par excellence
for resuscitation.)

(1) Atropine sulphate for vagal inhibition and

sinus slowing.

(2) Caffeine citrate or aminophyllin for acute pulmonary edema or respiratory stimulant.

(3) Calcium chloride for the refractory stage of epinephrine.

(4) Hexamethonium for hypertensive crisis and acute pulmonary edema.

(5) Quinidine for ventricular tachycardia and ventricular premature beats. (Intravenously with extreme caution.)

(6) Mephentermine, neosynephrine, levo-nor-epinephrine (levophed), vasopressors, which have been alluded to already. These are to be employed for hypotension which is not due to blood loss or arrhythmias.

(7) Hydrocortisone sodium succinate to restore sensitivity of the vascular bed to vasopressors.

(8) Lantoside C (Cedilanid) for myocardial failure.

When the patient is recovering from this disaster, his condition must be evaluated carefully to detect cardiac abnormalities. These disturbances, especially disorders of rhythm, are usually diagnosed by a cardiologist with the aid of an electrocardiogram. Supraventricular arrhythmias are usually innocuous. A standby pacemaker may prove useful.

Secretions should be removed early by tracheal and bronchial aspiration. In those who are semicomatose, aspiration may be necessary every fifteen to thirty minutes. If these secretions are well taken care of there will be a minimum occurrence of post-operative atelectasis. A tracheostomy set should be on hand. This important life saving* procedure has not been used early enough or frequently enough.

Pneumothorax with its resultant dyspnea can be corrected by careful aspiration of the pleural space.

If there is cardio-respiratory embarrassment from effusion, remove the excessive fluid by aspiration.

Failure of the lung to expand may be due to several causes, the simplest being failure to change the position of the patient. Some of the other causes are: pneumothorax, hydrothorax, pulmonary edema, obstruction of the bronchus, irregular expansion of the lung causing loculations, and leakage around a drain. The obvious treatment is the removal of the cause.

A hematoma in the wound may be due to a bleeding intercostal vessel.

Wound infections are reduced to a minimum with the use of antibiotics despite the lack of sterile precautions.

When the patient is recovering from this disaster, his condition must be appraised carefully from minute to minute and he will need a great deal of

*Western European surgeons practiced tracheostomy in the 12th and 13th centuries.

attention and expert care. Without this, a successful resuscitation may have been done in vain.

BIBLIOGRAPHY

1. Seldon, T. H.: Postanesthetic Encephalopathy. *Staff Meet. Mayo Clinic, 24*:370, 1949.
2. Hosler, R. M.: Emergency Treatment of Cardiac Arrest. *J. Am. A. Nurse Anesth., 20*:18, 1952.

XVI

RESULTS

S EVERAL TYPES of results may be obtained.

(1) Full recovery of cerebral function, of respiration, and heart beat. This is the ideal result and the one that is hoped for.

(2) Full recovery of respiration and heart beat with delayed recovery of cerebral function, but eventual complete recovery. These patients may have a clouded sensorium for a short time or for several days. Convulsions may continue for several days also. Mollison[1] reported a patient remained unconscious for seven days and showed signs of cerebral irritation for a period of fourteen days. Permanent recovery ultimately occurred.

(3) Full recovery of respiration and heart beat, but permanent impairment of cerebral function. Fortunately this result does not occur frequently. The majority of these people either completely recover or expire, (1% estimated).

(4) Full recovery of the heart beat and blood pressure, but delay in the recovery of normal respiration. Bohn[2] reported a case in which the normal respiratory function was not obtained until two and

one-half hours following the return of a cardiac rhythm.

(5) Temporary recovery of heart beat, but gradual decrease of blood pressure and death within two to twelve hours in spite of all measures to sustain blood pressure.

(6) Full recovery of respiration and heart beat, but death from cerebral edema on the following day or succeeding days.

(7) Recovery of heart beat without recovery of respiration; the heart continues to beat only as long as mechanical respiration is administered.

(8) Inability to restore the heart beat. This is usually due to poor resuscitation technique or inherent cardiac disease. In those unsuccessful cases, I believe it to be a good policy to have the anesthetist and a hospital representative accompany the surgeon at the time that the family is informed of this misfortune.

In the study of successful cases one is impressed with the superiority of results of those cases in which the chest was already open when the heart ceased to beat. Massage could at once be undertaken. The factor of time of arrest was practically removed and the factor of indecision had been eliminated.

BIBLIOGRAPHY

1. Mollison, W. M.: Heart Massage Through Abdominal Incision. *Brit. J. Chest Dis., 14*:42, 1917.
2. Bohn, G. L.: *Brit. M. J., 2*:725, 1939.

XVII

FIELDS OF APPLICATION

THE SCOPE of this life saving procedure is enlarging and new dimensions are being added. Yet, resuscitation is still in its infancy. Experience leads us to believe, resuscitation may under satisfactory circumstances be effectually applied to victims in these additional categories.

1. Acute coronary insufficiency with "mechanism death."
2. Electrocution.
3. Drowning.
4. Heart block.
5. Asphyxia.
6. Paralysis of respiratory center.
   drugs,
   poliomyelitis
7. Massive hemorrhage.
8. Acute carbon monoxide poisoning and other noxious gases.
9. Cardiac catheterization.
10. Hypotensive surgery.
11. Air embolism.
12. New-born infants.

13. Anaphylaxis.

14. Impending death from exposure to extreme cold.

15. Possibly in well-organized dental offices.

16. Possibly in well-organized power stations.

Brevity precludes a detailed discussion of all the above categories. However, it can be readily seen that the general principles as outlined in this book are applicable to those victims. The requirements are that trained personnel reach the victim within the time limitation following cessation of an effectual circulation, and that the proper equipment is available. Some lives will thus be saved. How many, only further developments will determine.

To quote from Paluel J. Flagg, "A curious and unfortunate situation has accompanied the evolution of resuscitation in the United States. The layman has been so far in advance of the physician in his contact with the patient, not only physically but in his First-Aid interest, that resuscitation has become identified with lay relief. This identification of resuscitation with lay services has brought about a double effect, which has served to retard a serious professional approach to the problem. On one hand the physician has come to regard resuscitation as something beneath his professional attention, and on the other the rescue squad has come to look upon the asphyxiated patient as its exclusive problem to which the physician has little if anything to contribute.

"To add to the confusion, manufacturers of resuscitation apparatus have flooded the field with mechanical robots, each fortified with by unimpeachable scientific research quite unintelligible to the prospective purchasers. Indeed, this scientific support for mechanical devices for resuscitation equipment has reached a point where the average physician asked to pass judgment upon their relative merits is bewilderd by the claims which he is asked to adjudicate by virture of his medical education. Such a physician finds himself in a position in which he is asked to act upon a medical problem for which his medical-school training did not fit him, for asphyxia as a major medical problem and the scientific means of relief attracted little attention.

All physicians have a strong obligation to educate themselves in the principles of recognizing and treating hypoxia. The medical schools and hospitals of the nation should provide leadership."

The future undoubtedly holds some promise for those whom fate has been generous enough to grant a fatal "heart attack" in a location where personnel trained in resuscitation and the proper equipment is on hand. Our conception of so-called death must necessarily undergo new consideration for the death factor at times is reversible.

ACUTE CORONARY INSUFFICIENCY WITH MECHANISM DEATH

At this moment the above statement will not be universally accepted, but will the future regard the following extra-ordinary incident (case number VIII) commonplace?[1]

On June 22, 1955, a 65 year old practicing physician of Cleveland collapsed on the floor, near the hospital's emergency ward. This doctor had precordial pain the previous day and no doubt had recently had a coronary occlusion. Only a few minutes before his collapse an electrocardiogram had been taken.

Two surgeons were behind him and they carried him to the nearby accident room, where adequate help and equipment were available. He was cyanosed, had no pulse nor respiration. There were no heart sounds. Oxygen was administered by a face mask, and without hesitation or delay his shirt was ripped off and within three to four minutes his heart was being massaged and his lungs ventilated. Shortly thereafter an intratracheal tube was inserted. The heart was in coarse ventricular fibrillation, and after several strong shocks of 3 amperes were delivered, it returned to a coordinated beat. In a relative short time his blood pressure and pulse returned to normal. He was successfully resuscitated with his shoes and trousers on. His post-resuscitative course was uncomplicated except for a clouded sensorium for a few days and a slight wound infection.

One feature apt to be overlooked is that this incident dramatically and emphatically demonstrates that a small amount of oxygenated blood represents the difference between life and death in coronary insufficiency. Usually it is a problem of unequal distribution in the myocardium rather than the amount available. In this instance, manipulation and surface excoriation greatly effected this delicate balance, so that after three months this man returned to the practice of medicine and some two years later is in good health.

Resuscitation is now feasible in those people

facing impending death from acute coronary insufficiency, if the victim dies in the hospital. Preparation for such a procedure should be made before
death occurs. This should consist of having a mobile
emergency resuscitation cart outside of his room and
a precise, mental rehearsal by the team. Otherwise, a
frantic inefficient atmosphere may prevail during the
exigency. Grouping of these "coronary" patients in
convenient areas of the hospital is suggested.

ELECTROCUTION

Death from electrocution ordinarily results
from ventricular fibrillation or paralysis of the respiratory center. As has been already emphasized on
page 103, moderately weak currents as used in the
home can be extremely hazardous if the person is
well grounded. This can result in instantaneous
death due to ventricular fibrillation. The victim is
pulseless. Artificial respiration cannot remedy this
condition.

Electro-convulsive therapy and its modifications
carry a small but significant case fatality rate. This
rate, which, however, is not precisely known has been
estimated to be in the order of one death per 1000
patients treated. Most of these procedures are carried
out with voltages between 130 and 140.

Electrocution by stronger currents and extremely high voltages cause contractions of the muscles
preventing breathing and at the same time it can

cause respiratory center paralysis. However, this amount of current prevents ventricular fibrillation. At the moment the current is broken the heart is defibrillated. This may not result in death. If there is any indication of a pulse, mechanical respiration can be undertaken. The respiratory center may only be temporarily paralyzed.

Powerful muscular contractions from strong currents may throw the victim free from the source of the shock. This is fortunate as only a split second shock may have been received, still it can be enough to paralyze the respiratory center. In other instances the person cannot be removed from the wire unless the current is broken. Under these circumstances the most expedient way may be to pry him loose with a wooden pole or throw a heavy coat around a foot and attempt to pull him loose. Care must be taken to insulate the rescuer.

Current is the killing factor in electrical shock. The voltage is important only in that it determines how much current will flow through a given body of resistance. We know from laboratory* experience that a small amount of current can cause ventricular fibrillation while it takes a strong current to defibrillate the animals' hearts.

EDISON ELECTRIC INSTITUTE — INDUSTRY REPORT
ELECTROCUTIONS FOR 1955 FROM ELECTRIC POWER COMPANIES

Volts	Cases	Resuscitated	Died	% Saved
110-480	12	1	11	8
2000-3000	34	9	25	26
6000-8000	22	8	14	34

*In our laboratory we use 25 milli-amperes to cause fibrillation in the dog's heart. To defibrillate this same heart we use 2.5 amperes.

DROWNING

Insurance statistics indicate that over 6000 civilians drown each year in these United States. In the Armed Services during the period from 1942 to 1953, 8,065 lives were lost due to drowning. This figure represented twenty-five per cent of all non-battle casualties.

Drowning may be defined as suffocation in a liquid such as water. It is reasonable to consider that drowning has been a common mode of accidental death since antiquity. It probably constitutes the most common type of asphyxia. Early medical writers gave this subject a great deal of attention. It is apparent that the 18th century writers were becoming aware of the various aspects of asphyxia.

Often the victim[2] in the act of drowning becomes hysterical, cries out, and struggling may last for two minutes. In ten per cent, laryngeal spasm may be acute and no water is found in the lungs. In ninety per cent of cases, huge amounts of water are gulped and found in the stomach. This in turn induces vomiting with aspiration of water, leading to asphyxia.

The temperature and the type of the water greatly influences many of the important time factors. In fresh water, drowning often leads to cardiac arrest in two to four minutes. In salt water this often leads to cardiac cessation in six to seven minutes.

Fresh water rapidly passes through the alveolar

membrane into the blood stream causing hemodilution. Within three minutes, more than seventy per cent of the circulating body fluid may be composed of fresh water with instantaneous and critical lowering of the blood electrolytes. Too often this results in potassium intoxication which induces ventricular fibrillation. The additional potassium is released from erythrocytes which are rapidly hemolyzed.

Following suffocation in *sea water, there is marked and rapid hemo-concentration of the circulating blood. There is little change in the potassium to sodium ion ratio. Plasma proteins diffuse into the alveolar bed with resultant pulmonary edema and overwhelming anoxia. In the meantime the heart is functioning as a pump to the best of its ability. At the same time small but significant amounts of oxygen are being removed from muscle groups and transported to the heart and brain. These organs have the ability to wring out the so-called last drop of oxygen. Depending upon the circumstances it is reasonable to assume that people have been successfully resuscitated after ten minutes. If death supervenes, it occurs as a result of anoxic myocardial failure.

Ordinary resuscitative efforts will fail if one is ABSOLUTELY certain there is no pulse. Do not waste time trying to prove or disprove this fact. Some

---

*Sea water has 3.5% Na cl.

form of artificial respiration must be started at once. Of course 100 per cent oxygen delivered by alternate pressure on a bag[3] is preferred (Figure 17). The person should be placed on his abdomen with the head at a lower level. Make sure there is no blockage of the airway from foreign material or vomitus.

For those nearly drowned in fresh water, venesection and 3-5 per cent sodium chloride solution intravenously is indicated. If the medium is salt water, sterile water or 5 per cent glucose is given intravenously as well as other supporting measures.

HEART BLOCK

Complete heart block refers to the unique inherent rhythmic characteristic of a heart muscle. A slow somewhat irregular rhythm is typical. This is called idio-ventricular rhythm. There is a complete dissociation between the auricular and ventricular rates. After the heart rate slows to a certain point, it becomes ineffectual in sustaining a satisfactory blood pressure and circulation. The patient will then suffer a syncopal attack. Clinically, this is most frequently seen in the Stokes-Adams Syndrome, which is not a surgical disease.

The external artificial pacemaker or heart pacer* finds its greatest application in this condition. These electrical instruments operate from conventional current. Electrodes are similar to those used in

*Figure 15, pg. 166.

electrocardiography. Good contact is assured with electrode paste. One electrode is placed over the apex of the heart, while considerable latitude exists in the placing of the other electrode. The frequency of pulses is usually variable between fifty and one hundred-fifty per minute. Their amplitude is adjustable between 0-130 volts. Only attentive alertness will insure against interruption of stimuli. Electrical provisions are available which will allow the instrument to remain in constant operation while the patient is being transported and is thus away from a wall socket.

It is generally agreed that in order for this artificial stimulator to produce a cardiac output it must be applied not later than 1 minute after complete arrest. (This is the maximum time).

It is my opinion that the pacemaker has not found a proper niche in resuscitation of surgical patients (page 103). It has no value in ventricular fibrillation. In the post-resuscitative period it can bolster a slow irregular faltering heart beat.

ASPHYXIA

Over two thousand years have elapsed since Aristotle made the observation that breathing was difficult on Mount Olympus because the air was too thin. Down through the ages man has come to have a much better understanding of the problems of asphyxia (see page 8). Only within the past few decades has intensive research been devoted to determining some of the specific effects of lack of oxygen on the brain. As of today, beyond the middle of the twentieth century, resuscitation is still in its early stage of development.

Asphyxia may be designated as histoxic, anemic, stagnant, and anoxic. The first three act slowly, but are insidious; they are dangerous because they may be overlooked.

PARALYSIS OF RESPIRATORY CENTER

Extreme respiratory depression and circulatory depression terminating in respiratory paralysis may result from overdosage or excessive amounts of anesthesia, alcohol, opiates, barbiturates, or electrical shock. Actually this is an incomplete list, but portrays the general picture.

Victims of acute anterior poliomyelitis have been resuscitated after succumbing from asphyxiation either from obstruction of the airway due to the accumulation of mucous and secretions or from the bulbar effects of the disease. The oxygen system was re-established by clearing the airway, (Endotracheal intubation or tracheostomy) mechanical respiration, and thoracotomy.

AIR EMBOLISM

My first introduction to cardiac arrest took place during my internship in 1933. A healthy young woman had sudden cessation of her circulation from air embolism resulting from a simple Rubin's test under anesthesia. After ten minutes of useless compressing of the thoracic cage and the injection of stimulants, Claude Beck was called. Oxygen was administered by a face mask and a thoracotomy was quickly done. The heart resumed a satisfactory beat after a short period of massage. This was the first time that I had seen or even heard of this procedure being carried out on a human. The patient died some eighteen hours later of cerebral edema.

The threat of air embolism is becoming more prevalent, i.e., open cardiac surgery; intravenous therapy and nutrition, rapid changes of atmospheric pressure under various conditions.

Nowadays it is recommended that if air embolism were suspected, aspiration of the right ventricular chamber could be quickly carried out with a needle and 20 cc. syringe before manual massage were instituted.

ACUTE CARBON MONOXIDE POISONING

Its extreme toxicity is due to the fact that its affinity for hemoglobin is 210 times greater than that of oxygen.

On occasions victims of acute carbon* monoxide poisoning reach the hospital in the stage where

---

*Cytochrome C is recommended intravenously in doses of 15-60 mg.

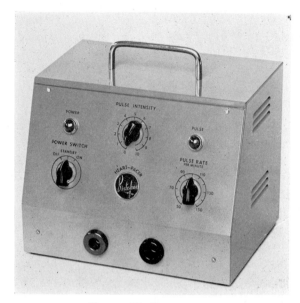

FIGURE 15. Heartpacer.

impending respiratory paralysis and death are imminent. Successful resuscitation may be possible with oxygen delivered into the lungs and replacement of a large percentage of the blood volume. If cardiac arrest should supervene at any juncture, direct handling of the heart is indicated.

NEW-BORN INFANTS

Serious attempts to resuscitate new-born infants dates back to the middle of the eighteenth century. During the first half of the nineteenth century, great interest in this particular field is noted. However, it seems that practically none of their methods have stood the test of time. The concept introduced by Little in 1842 that many physical disabilities in children are attributable to asphyxia in the new born was forgotten and had to be learned all over again.

Asphyxia in the new-born warrants deliberate exposure of their airway. Suction is immediately applied to relieve any offending secretions. The patency must be determined. Direct intubation under vision is followed by the insufflation of oxygen.

BIBLIOGRAPHY

1. Beck, C. S., *et al.*: Fatal Heart Attack. Successful Defibrillation. *J.A.M.A., 161:*434, 1956.
2. Swann, H. G.: Drowning. *Tex. Rep., Biol. & Med.,* 5:423, 1947.
3. Hingson, R. A.: Portable Resuscitator. *J.A.M.A., 156:* 604, 1954.

XVIII

THE COURSE IN CARDIAC RESUSCITATION

IN JANUARY, 1950, Doctors Beck, Rand and Hosler began formulating plans to initiate a short course in resuscitative principles. The Cleveland Area Heart Society supplied a grant of money. A few local institutions were approached, but they felt that there would not be enough interest to warrant a course.

After 10 months of planning and considering the site, the Cleveland Area Heart Society inaugurated its first course in Cardiac Resuscitation on November 9th, 1950. It was exceptionally well received and has become a monthly educational program for anesthetists and surgeons. To date, almost 1450 enthusiastic participants have taken the two-day course and they have been from the four corners of the United States as well as some from Europe, South America, Mexico, and Canada. Two courses were given in 1952 at the Army Medical Service Graduate School at Walter Reed Army Medical Center in Washington, D. C. The Cleveland Area Heart Society has its office at 1689 East 115th Street, Cleveland, Ohio and continues to handle the applications.

The classes are informal and practical. Each participant has been asked the question as to whether or not he has ever actually seen ventricular fibrillation in the human or in the laboratory animal. The number that have had this experience varies from twenty to forty per cent. The term cardiac arrest on the operating table was more or less universally unheard of during academic years. In general the belief that the cause of cardiac arrest is unknown was accepted by many.

The initial class sessions include introductory and explanatory lectures and movies. This is followed by aseptic animal experiments. In the first of these experiments, the heart is permitted to stop in standstill or asystole, by a breakdown of the oxygen system for a period longer than the safe time limit. In the second experiment, the heart is placed into ventricular fibrillation by an electrical shock for a period of two minutes. These animals are revived and then observed the following day. The results are impressive and dramatic. The impression is long lasting.

The afternoon (session) is concerned with lectures in predisposing factors and danger signals leading up to cardiac arrest. These have been given by Doctor Robert Hingson and staff. Lectures and demonstrations at the laboratory table on the physiology of the heart beat and the role of cardiac drugs

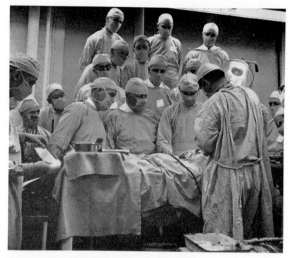

FIGURE 16. Cleveland Cardiac Resuscitation Class in action. Doctor Beck is standing on opposite side of table, second from left to right. (Photo reproduced by permission of *The Saturday Evening Post*.)

are given by Doctor Frederick R. Mautz.

The highlight of the course is the final session on the following day during which time the class members are given an opportunity to practice cardiac massage. Each member produces cardiac arrest and then institutes a coordinated effectual heart beat.

The various means and methods of massage are carried out in such a way that each member can observe his own technique as he watches a continuous writing and recording of the effective blood pressure that he is sustaining. It is interesting to note the improvement of the blood pressure with the improvement of the massage technique. No member is permitted to finish the class until he has brought the heart out of ventricular fibrillation at least once. Usually one animal suffices for this session. The animal's heart is brought out of fibrillation at least twenty to twenty-eight times. We have more or less taken for granted the fact that the laboratory animal's heart can be stopped and restored to a normal rhythm at will. This is a non-sterile experiment and at the end of the exercise the animal is sacrificed.

In 1954 the Cleveland Area Heart Society sent out a questionnaire pertaining to this course. Out of 500 questionnaires sent, 276 replied. Among the successful cases reported were two physicians, one of international reputation. This total of 44* is no doubt greater, for there are many unreported cases. The data collected by means of this questionnaire, as shown in the table, reveal pertinent facts concerning the value of preparedness and planning for such disasters. It appears that cardiac arrest is not a rarity, since thirty-one per cent of the group who answered the questionnaire had occasion to treat patients with this condition after they had taken the course. It is encouraging to know that 74.6 per cent of the group who took the course are now working in hospitals

*This figure of 44 successful cases has now pyramided.

where an organized program is being carried out.

SUMMARY OF 276 REPLIES TO THE
QUESTIONNAIRE ON CARDIAC RESUSCITATION

Question	Yes	No	Un-answered
1. Have you had occasion to use resuscitation procedures since taking this course?	85	191	0
2. If so, were you successful?	44	35	6
3. Do you find that knowledge in this subject helped prevent possible disaster?	235	19	22
4. Does your hospital have an organized program for the prevention and management of cardiac arrest?	206	52	18

The results of this survey indicate that patients today may suffer from cardiac arrest during the induction of the anesthesia, during the actual operation, or immediately following it. But an expert team that knows what to do and how to use the necessary equipment can save many of these patients.

By March 1, 1956,* 1000 had participated in this course in the prevention and management of cardiac arrest, which had originated as an orphan. Geographically they had come from thirty-four different states in the U.S.A. Some of the foreign countries included: Canada, Brazil, Spain, Phillipines, England, Venezuela, Switzerland, Puerto Rico, Cuba, Guatemala, Belgium, Ecuador, Mexico, Scotland, Argentina, Formosa, Japan, France, and Germany.

The recipients of university degrees from numerous schools in thirty-one separate foreign countries

---

*By June 1957, 1400 participants.

are included in the participation group.

One comment from the Chief of a Surgical Service in referring to the Course was as follows: "The mental attitude engendered, which prepares the surgeon for instant action, will save many lives through elimination of hesitation and vacillation."

A few of the reports of interesting and educational cases follows:

Case I. Patient, age 52. Operated, July 2, 1952. Gastric resection for bleeding duodenal and gastric ulcer, about one-third completed when cardiac arrest occurred. Prompt thoracotomy revealed cardiac tamponade, hemopericardium from perforated left ventricle at site of myocardial infarct (probably a week preceding the operation and unsuspected). Blood removed. Heart massaged. Given intracardiac procaine and adrenalin. Repaired myocardial blowout with mattress sutures and gelfoam. Closed chest and then completed the subtotal resection. Electrocardiogram showed myocardial infarct, now six days post-operatively. He is making a satisfactory recovery.*

C. W. McNamara, M.D.

Case II. Patient, age 5. Patient had had recurrent attacks of septic tonsillitis for three years and it was decided that a tonsillectomy and adenoidectomy

---

*Later expired in Hospital (personal communication).

was indicated. On November 1, 1951, 1/300th grain of atropine was given at eight o'clock. Gas and oxygen anesthesia was given to the patient followed by drop ether and later by ether with the suction machine. The operation was performed without any difficulty whatsoever. The patient made an uneventful recovery. On November 6, 1951, the patient returned at eight o'clock in the morning complaining of bleeding at the nose for four hours duration. The patient seemed to be in good shape and had not lost too much blood. Adrenalin packs were inserted in the nose and the patient was put to bed in the hospital. At 9:30 that morning through consultation it was decided that the bleeding was coming from the adenoid area, and it was advisable to re-anesthetize the patient and pack the adenoid area. 1/300th grain of atropine was given fifteen minutes before the beginning of the anesthesia with gas and oxygen. About the time that the patient was considered to be under surgical anesthesia there was some gurgling in the patient's throat. A mouth gag was inserted in the mouth and a large clot had slipped down from the adenoid area in the region of the epiglottis. This clot was removed quickly with a sponge forcep. The patient began to wake up and in the meantime became cyanotic. Palpation of the heart over the chest area showed it to be very slow and it beat only a few times before it ceased beating. Oxygen was immediately applied by compression upon the oxygen bag.

After three minutes by my watch the chest was entered and the heart was at complete standstill. The pericardium was opened and the heart was massaged manually and a half cubic centimeter of adrenalin chloride was injected into the right heart chamber. The heart was massaged for forty-five minutes without any response. Upon opening the chest the left lung was completely collapsed. We did not have any method for intratracheal intubation. Some of the oxygen that was pumped through the bag had entered the stomach.*

M.D.

Case III. Patient, white physician, age 83. Exploration of abdomen for incarcerated inguinal hernia under N_2O-O_2, ether, endotracheal. Anesthesia course normal. Blood pressure normal until manipulation of distended loops of bowel. In spite of proper plane of surgical anesthesia, the blood pressure dropped to zero and there was cardiac arrest. Cardiac massage immediately instituted brought back the blood pressure to a normal reading. Respiration returned, the operation was completed and the patient made an uneventful convalescence.

F. A. SMITH, M.D.

*Author's note: Failure was probably due to inability to carry out oxygenation. If intubation were not possible, tracheotomy and the introduction of a rubber tube might have been beneficial. There also may have been blockage of the left mainstem bronchus by a clot. There was an obvious reduction of hemoglobin.

Case IV. Patient was admitted to Toledo Hospital on February 14, 1952 with a diagnosis of spontaneous rupture of the esophagus. The patient was prepared for thoracotomy. In the operating room anesthesia was induced with intravenous pentothal and an endotracheal tube was inserted. Immediately after the tube had been placed in the trachea, the anesthetist noticed that the patient was in cardiac arrest. The anesthetist started artificial respiration by rhythmical pressure on the anesthetic bag. No pulse was palpable for a period of 60 seconds. An incision was made rapidly through the left anterior chest through the fifth intercostal space. The hand was inserted through the pleural cavity and the heart was palpated through the pericardium. The heart was flabby. There was no contraction. It was massaged for a period of about sixty seconds. Regular contractions started and a normal heart beat resumed. The heart massage was instituted roughly about two minutes after cardiac arrest was noted.

The patient was then turned on the right lateral recumbent position and a planned thoracotomy and repair of ruptured esophagus was carried out. This procedure took about two hours. The heart beat remained normal throughout the operation. The patient made an uneventful recovery and has remained well to date.

M. W. SELMAN, M.D.

Case V. Twice during decortication of a constrictive pericarditis, cardiac standstill occurred and each time it responded well to massage, the first time after about one minute of massage and the second time after four minutes of massage. The case was successful.

J. H. WALKER, M.D.

Case VI. The notable case of the successful resuscitation of a student nurse in Chicago is a singular example of good judgment. While the surgeon massaged the fibrillating heart, thus keeping up an effective circulation to the vital organs, the Beck-Rand Defibrillating machine was brought across the town from another hospital by police escort and then applied successfully. One individual carried out the major portion of the manual massage and found his forearm swollen and tired the next day.

1951

Case VII. Patient, a 62 year old internationally known cardiologist, was to undergo a right upper lobectomy for minimal tuberculous lesion. Pre-operation medication consisted of Seconal, 100 mg. at 6:30 a.m. and Demerol, 75 mg. and Scopolamine, .6 mg. at 8:00 a.m. Induction was begun at 8:27 with sodium pentothal. At 8:36 an attempt was made to introduce an endotracheal tube. The patient coughed and induction was continued. At 8.42 there was recognized peripheral vascular collapse. At 8:43 the patient was intubated. At 8:44 there was cardiac slowing; atropine .8 mg. was given intravenously. At 8:45 arrest was recognized. Massage through left thoracotomy was begun at 8:46½.

By 9:02, after the use of .5cc. of 1/20,000 adrenalin, cardiac action was fair but assisted massage was necessary. There then occurred a perforation of the right ventricle through a paper thin scar resulting from previous known coronary thrombosis. This perforation was sutured after great difficulty and considerable loss of blood. Massage was continued but cardiac action was never strong enough to maintain circulation despite the repeated use of adrenalin and calcium chloride. Ventricular fibrillation never supervened. Finally, after more than three hours and fifty minutes of massage, satisfactory cardiac action was obtained, aided by peripheral vasoconstrictors, and the chest was closed.

The patient remained in the operating room. During the evening he recovered consciousness and showed no sign of mental deterioration. He continued to improve without evidence of damage to the brain, liver or kidneys. However, he had had an increase in his tuberculosis and has remained in cardiac failure, more or less controlled despite his return home.   H. SLOAN, M.D.

Case VIII. This case is reported in detail on page 156. This physician "dropped dead" of a coronary attack on June 22, 1955. He would have remained dead and been buried had he not been resuscitated.

Three months later he returned to his practice and worked over eight months before retiring. I spent one morning with him at the 1957 A.M.A. exhibition hall and am pleased to report he is more active than I am. He has taken only one nitro since "his operation" and states emphatically: "I am very happy the attempt was made."

It would appear that the "death factor" in this instance was definitely of a minor magnitude. This type of successful resuscitation will follow the same pattern of successful resuscitation in the operating room subsequent to anesthesia. The feasibility of this procedure to change one's condition from temporary death to one of living is gradually being proved. At times only a fine thread separates death from future living in this world.

A 42 years old male was admitted to the Sisters of Charity Hospital in Buffalo on June 17, 1957 with a diagnosis of acute myocardial infarction. His room was directly across from the nurse's station. About six hours after admission, respiration and pulse suddenly ceased. Artificial respiration and the application of an oxygen mask failed to clear up the cyanosis.

Several minutes later the chest was opened with scissors. Massage was instituted through the intact pericardium which was followed by a radial pulse and improvement in the patient's color. Forty-five minutes later a strong ventricular fibrillation was obvious. Two counter shocks at this time returned the heart to a coordinated beat and resulted in an effective circulation. A massive posterior wall infarct was demonstrated by the electrocardiogram. The patient remained in a coma for over two days. There was a gradual, but complete clearing of the central nervous system which took a period of three months. He returns to active work on November 1, 1957. He exhibits only a loss of memory for the three weeks following cardiac arrest. This successful resuscitative procedure was managed in the patient's room.

(Reported to author by Drs. Edward Kopf, Floyd Zaepel, and Joseph J. Roberts on October 14, 1957).

XIX

OXYGEN, THE FUEL OF LIFE

ROBERT A. HINGSON, M.D.

Professor Anesthesia, School of Medicine, Western Reserve University and Director of Anesthesia, University Hospitals of Cleveland.

RESPIRATORY resuscitation, its knowledge and technic is far more important in the front-line rescue team who reach the victims in the precious moments of salvage than in the physician and hospital team who usually get to the victims minutes to hours later when the "die is already cast." In Hiroshima, Father Siemes reported that thirty hours after the explosion elapsed before organized rescue parties were observed. In fact, 90 per cent of the doctors and 1654 out of 1780 nurses were killed by the blast and only three civilian hospitals were left standing.

It is our belief that this knowledge of rescue at present is sparsely and inadequately distributed even among those who should know it best and who are confronted with victims most frequently in rapid transit from salvageable humans to the state of the "corpus delecti." Therefore we think a review of the principles of maintaining oxygenation and respiration is timely for every thinking person who at some time in life, and perhaps today, will have an opportunity to save a life—and, more important, a brain in the life of a salvageable victim—whether it be beside the crib of an infant with whooping cough, croup or asthma, or at the swimming pool, a burning hotel or at the awful periphery of an atomic blast.

Remember, at sea level uncontaminated air contains 20 per cent oxygen. At least 500cc. or one pint of air must enter the lungs and leave the lungs 12 to 20 times each minute. Within 2 to 5 minutes from the time the victim's supply is cut off death ensues. Supply this need by the following rules:

1. Be calm; act purposefully and promptly; THINK!

2. Clear the entire airway from nose and mouth to the throat, of water, blood, vomit or foreign body by finger, absorbent cloth or suction apparatus.

3. Let gravity help by placing head down, body up on inclined plane or simply holding infant or child up by ankles.

4. Apply artificial respiration by the most effective method you best understand.

a) The oldest and still effective one is that used by Elisha in the Bible, II Kings 4:34, mouth to mouth alternate blowing and releasing. Thousands* of infants have been saved in this manner in times

---

*Authors' note: Kaiser Wilhelm II, was kept alive by a peasant nurse maid after the physicians who had delivered him gave up.

past by physicians and midwives. One of the Dionne quintuplets was kept alive for more than an hour by this method. Likewise, suction through a metal or rubber tube or even a paper straw by the rescue operator will clear the throat and mouth of a victim.

b) The prone Schafer method.

c) The alternate open palm compression and release of the upper front (anterior) part of the chest.

d) The arm life–hand squeeze of lower rib cage.

Alternate inflation and deflation of the chest with positive pressure air or oxygen saves lives. This can be accomplished by either the Kreiselman, Evans, E. & J., Ohio Chemical or Mines Safety artificial ventilators, if one of them is available and its operation is understood by the rescue team. However, these complicated machines have often been the decoys that have lost time and life and brain also, through menacing mechanical failure and mask leaks, with too much focus of attention on such heavy, expensive machines (and sometimes inaccessible) that even baffle more than half the doctors who try to use them. All of these methods take skill, practice, and visual and audible verification of effectiveness. We are not satisfied with these methods in many cases, even though they must be used and are life-saving in many others. In our Departments of Anesthesia at Western Reserve University of Cleveland, Ohio, and in former departments of the primary author in U. S. Marine Hospitals, on warships at sea, and in the Departments of Anesthesia at Jefferson University, University of Tennessee and Johns Hopkins Hospital, a constant effort has been made for twenty-five years to improve existing apparatus and technic.

On a sunny morning, August 6th, 1945, 120,000 people were killed or later died of injuries from the A-Bomb at Hiroshima. At Texas City, Texas, a cargo ship loaded with nitrites and twine exploded, killing 560 and injuring 4800, with widespread smoke, fires and burns. The San Francisco earthquake in 1906 left behind 452 dead and a city swept by fire. Even more devastating was the 1923 earthquake in Japan that killed 99,331 and injured 103,733. In the famous Cleveland Clinic fire twenty-seven years ago, there was little flame above the basement, yet 125 victims died from smoke poisoning. The Metropolitan Life Insurance Company reports that drowning, which is the third largest cause of accidental death, claims 6500 lives per year in the United States. The most important single factor in the treatment of drowning is artificial respiration. More than twice as many die from asphyxia than from automobile accidents. Such a recital could continue indefinitely. Disasters strike in many forms, but all combine certain common salient features.

1. They are frequently unheralded.
2. Medical personnel is overburdened and medi-

cal supplies are usually inadequate. Emergency mobile hospital units may be necessary with the administration of modified treatment.

3. Help from the outside is usually slow in forming.

4. Large scale panics invariably inhibit effective emergency action.

To cope with these problems, the government of the United States has supervised the establishment of numerous emergency teams of medical and civilian personnel, among them the Civilian Defense. It is the objective of these teams that they will stand organized and ready to supply the necessary help required to prevent and alleviate the panic, the transmission of infectious diseases, the spread of fires and destruction; and to facilitate help from outside of the disaster area.

Since the advent of atomic warfare, for the first time since the Revolutionary War an enemy has the ability to threaten our nation's existence. It thus behooves every citizen to be prepared in the event of any disaster, whether it be during peace or war, to remain clearheaded in order to move and act in the direction which will help himself and others around him.

In this discussion the author wishes to discuss the role that oxygen and artificial ventilation play in medical care during emergencies. Every year 6500 persons in this country die from drowning and 1300 die from gas asphyxia and about 40,000 in railway and automobile accidents. It would be foolish to even estimate the number of persons that could be saved every year by prompt and proper administration of oxygen. In Miami, Florida, which averages 2200 fires per year, there hasn't been a man knocked out by fumes since 1949. They have been able to maintain their remarkable record by the timely use of self-contained oxygen equipment. Certainly this is good firemanship in view of the fact that 5000 to 6000 firemen are felled by fumes every year.

FUNDAMENTAL CONSIDERATIONS

The pair of human lungs in the normal adult with a total maximum capacity of about one gallon of free volume air is charged with the responsible function of transmitting 4 teaspoonfuls (20 cc.) of oxygen each breath from surface exposure to the oxygen-hungry pulmonary capillary blood stream en route to the left side of the heart. Of almost equal importance is the lungs' discharge each breath of 4 teaspoonsfuls (20 cc.) of carbon dioxide en route from the body's carburetor to the exhaled air. By day and night as long as life lasts this function is repeated 12 to 20 times per minute at rest and 30 to 60 times a minute during heavy exercise and periods of rapid body growth. In all, about 70 square meters of lung membrane more delicate than fine silk are involved in this exchange. Seven hundred and fifty million air sacs (alvoeli) embrace micro-pockets of air and through partial pressure differential exchange carbon dioxide for oxygen or exchange the processes of potential death for the fuel of sustaining life. This phenomenon under normal circumstances cannot be interrupted more than two to four minutes without doing serious and even permanent damage to the three most vulnerable and important body organs: the brain, the heart, and the suprarenal gland.

As a dramatic example, a clamp completely compressing the trachea (windpipe) of a dozen rabbits, a dozen dogs, or a dozen humans for four minutes would result in unconsciousness, convulsions and heart standstill (death) in at least ten of the twelve and serious damage to the survivors. In diseases, infancy or old age the survival time would be of shorter duration.

To answer these demands as criteria of a resuscitation device, our research team in the fall of 1954 developed a new portable midget machine capable of providing an immediate supply of oxygen for resuscitation by inhalation for infants and adults (Figure 17). The machine weighs a little over one pound and is approximately two feet in length. A box of 24 cylinders (total of 72,000 cc. of pure oxygen) weighs 24 ounces.

Since its conception in 1954, there has been a continuous series of research projects concerning the

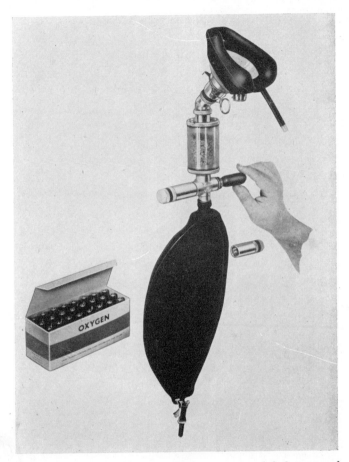

Figure 17. A portable resuscitator, oxygen inhalator, and anesthesia machine. Various gases are available in small cylinders. A small one pound unit, capable of performing life-saving functions.

machine, with the emphasis being placed on its usefulness as an inhalator and resuscitator. These studies were induced in an attempt to evaluate such factors as: 1) Proper size of the soda lime canister to maintain a safe carbon dioxide volume per cent in the rebreathed mixture; 2) length of time that the machine can be used as an inhalator-resuscitator under a variety of conditions such as walking, sitting, lying down, climbing steps, driving a car, et cetera. Oxygen consumption was also determined during these experiments. Gas samples were drawn into an evacuated tube from the rebreathing bag at periodic intervals and were analyzed on the Haldane-Boothby gas analyzer for carbon dioxide and oxygen percentage. To summarize these findings:

1) A young, non-fasting male adult walking at the rate of 3 miles per hour may use the machine to travel safely for:

    a. 200 yards using no canister
    b. 600 yards using 100 cc. canister
    c. 1100 yards using a 200 cc. canister
    d. 1800 yards using a 500 cc. canister

2) A young, nonfasting male adult in a sitting position may use the machine safely for:

    a. 2-3 minutes using no canister
    b. 15 minutes using a 100 cc. canister
    c. 60 minutes using a 200 cc. canister
    d. More than 60 minutes using a 500 cc. canister.

The temperature of the gases in the face mask ranged from 84°F. and never exceeded 100°F. throughout the course of the experiments.

In evaluating these results, it seems obvious that this machine is able to provide adequate oxygen in a convenient form for use under a variety of conditions both as an inhalator and a resuscitator. For example:

a. For the general practitioner. This device will readily fit into his bag and be immediately available for use either as an inhalator or resuscitator. It might also be mentioned that cylinders of cyclo-propane-helium and oxygen-helium are available for use in the machine to provide a non-explosive instantaneous anesthesia for short surgery, obstetrical deliveries, bone-setting, wound suturing or lancing of abscesses.

b. For the rescue squad, whether it be lay or professional. This device is small enough to fit into a man's pocket. By inflating and using positive hand pressure on the rebreathing bag an adequate amount of oxygen in amounts of 1000 cc. per hand squeeze is immediately made available in the lungs during resuscitation.

c. For the cardiac, asthmatic, emphysematous patient in transient respiratory distress. It is easy to operate, economical and convenient so that the patient may administer oxygen to himself as needed or upon the doctor's orders.

Technique for Use as a Resuscitator:

Position of the subject is important. He should be lying on his back in the Trendelenburg position. This serves two useful purposes: 1) Facilitates greater venous return, which aids in maintenance of blood pressure; 2) aids in the clearing of the lungs and bronchi of any foreign material which may, as a result of gravitational pull, run down into the oropharynx and nasopharynx instead of the trachea.

Before any attempt is ever made to resuscitate a victim, it is absolutely necessary that the airway to the lungs be unobstructed. Obstruction may be due to the presence of a foreign body, regurgitated gastric contents, relaxed tongue, or spasm of the larynx or bronchi. In case of the latter, suction and artificial airways are almost always necessary. The best way to insure an open airway through the oral cavity is by use of an oral rubber airway of the Guedel type, of the proper size. If this is not feasible, very often simple extension of the patient's head upon its axis will suffice to relieve pharyngeal obstruction, or by advancing the lower jaw forward by applying pressure to the back of the angles of the jaw. In cases of drowning where there is frequently water in the extra-pulmonary bronchi and even sometimes in the intrapulmonary bronchi, a useful device is a suction tube which can be run down the trachea to suck out the water. This is necessary since it is futile to administer oxygen to a patient without proper clearing of these air passages. If a suction tube is not handy, even soda straws may be substituted.

Having established a clear airway to the lungs, the machine is placed on the victim's face, making sure the mask fits snugly. The last two fingers of the left hand of the operator support the patient's jaw. The thumb, index and middle fingers cause downward pressure on the face mask. The operator's right hand compresses and releases the rubber bag rhythmically at about a rate of 12-15 times per minute. The amount of pressure exerted should be just enough to force oxygen into the subject's lungs, which would be a normal tidal volume, which can be visualized by observing chest expansion and deflation during the artificial respiratory cycle, remembering that there is a safety valve to prevent too much applied pressure from harming the subject.

If the machine is equipped with the 100cc. soda lime canister, resuscitation may be maintained for approximately 20 minutes, without danger of high carbon dioxide in the rebreathing mixture. However, if there is no fresh soda lime available it is certainly better to continue with the resuscitation in spite of the high carbon dioxide. It certainly would be better to insufflate the subject's lungs with oxygen containing less than 10 per cent carbon dioxide than no oxygen at all. The knowledge that carbon dioxide is much more depressing than such anesthetics as ethylene or nitrous oxide should prevent any consideration of using it to resuscitate unless it is necessary.

A supplementary technique is to remove the machine from the subject's face and empty the bag out completely, then refill it with pure oxygen, each five minutes. If the 200 cc. canister is used, the machine maybe used for periods of over one hour without danger of excess carbon dioxide effects. The 500 cc. canister can be used for 3-5 hours. In the case of lack of, or an inadequate supply of oxygen cylinders, the bag may be filled through the port in the end of the bag from larger oxygen cylinders or even by blowing short breaths into the port by the operator. If he can blow about 100 cc. of air into the bag with each breath, the subject will receive air with an oxygen content of about 20 per cent. The reason for this is that the first 130 cc. of expired air from a person is air that was unexposed to alveolar membranes and consequently has a composition exactly the same as that of atmospheric air.

If adequate cylinders are available, the operator should make sure that the bag is inflated at all times, i.e., as soon as the bag is half empty add another cylinder. This enables the operator to exert more efficient positive pressure on the bag as well as to keep down the carbon dioxide volumes per cent.

Removal of the machine should occur only when the subject shows clinical signs of recovery, i.e., normal respiratory rate and depth, normal pulse, and lack of any visible cyanosis or snycope.

The machine may be recommended for patients for self-adminstration as an inhalator, following the same rules of safe oxygen therapy as previously outlined.

DIFFERENCES IN CHILDREN AND ADULTS

Berglund, Gunilla, Karlberg and Petter in the Karolinska Institute in Stockholm have shown that the functional residual capacity (lung air after exhalation) of newborns is relatively two and one-half times lower than found in adults. This implies that an infant who has stopped breathing after exhalation is in several times greater danger than the adult since his reservoir of air is much less. Practically we have verified this important finding by observing that non-breathing infants and children become cyanotic (blue) much more rapidly than the adult. This indicates that even greater speed in resuscitation is required here—especially since the infants' metabolic requirement of oxygen is increased over that of adults.

Once breathing stops, the residual oxygen in the lung of a male adult patient who has exhaled after breathing air is only 16 per cent of 2000 cc. (2 quarts) or 320 cc.—less than a pint and less than four minutes from death. In contrast, the patient who has been breathing 100 per cent oxygen has two full quarts or at least a ten-minute supply before death.

The chances of saving life following asphyxia

from smoke, water, or the detonation of martial blast from noxious gas rests on a fleeting few precious minutes for the application of artificial ventilation by one of the methods mentioned above with pure air or preferably oxygen. The brain begins to die in the necessary and more fragile intelligence and memory centers first—then a few seconds later in the motor centers, to be swiftly followed by the heart itself. Oxygen sustains life. Oxygen saves life.

XX

LEGAL ASPECTS

I T WOULD BE FOLLY not to mention or consider the possibility of malpractice suits. It is difficult to understand how such an action could be drawn up against an alert surgeon who attempted resuscitation, but was unsuccessful. The primary question today is: Should the average surgeon be prepared to carry out cardiac resuscitative methods in his community? Should each hospital have the necessary equipment? That all surgeons have the necessary knowledge to carry out this resuscitative procedure and that all hospitals have the necessary equipment, are goals to be strived for. Achievement of these goals is something to be devoutly hoped for.

[1]Experience has taught that the most meticulous attention to the dictates of good medical practice is not sufficient to ward off the unjust claim, and that no physician is immune.

The physician must choose the method he will use. He may later wish he had selected another, and, in retrospect, perhaps a better method; but the physician must act without hindsight.

Malpractice has two essential parts: first, that

the physician fails to do his duty; and second, that definite injury to the patient is the result of his failure.

Any patient may bring a malpractice suit against any physician who has attended him professionally. The bringing of such an action does not, of course, even suggest that the claim has any merit.

No physician or surgeon[1] may be justifiably charged with malpractice unless, in the service rendered to his patient, he fails to meet the requirements of good professional practice, unless in the diagnosis or treatment of his patient, he omits to do something he should do or does something he should not do, measured against accepted standards of practice. The standard of practice is always what the ordinary reputable practitioner in the community, or similar communities, would do or would not do in the care of similar cases.

It is believed that the first malpractice suit in this field was taken to a court and jury in Cleveland, Ohio, on February 18, 1952. The plaintiff charged the surgeon with negligence for not attempting a cardiac resuscitative procedure. The hospital was charged with negligence for failure to have a stand-by surgeon who could open the patient's chest and carry out this procedure.

After two days of unprecedented charges and at the conclusion of the plaintiff's case, Judge Adrian Newcomb granted motions to arrest testimony and enter judgment FOR the defendants.

While no litigation on such a subject can be applauded, in this instance there may be considered to be beneficial results inasmuch as complacency was severely shaken up. Do not turn your back upon a cataclysmic disaster. Be prepared to keep the brain cells alive and keep out of the meshes of legal entanglements. Hesitation, vacillation, and indecision will have dynamic consequences. The resuscitative procedure is usually simple if one takes positive action. All that are necessary are:

> Courage
> Speed
> Clear Thinking
> Determination
> Perseverance
> A Few Special Instruments.

BIBLIOGRAPHY

1. Regan, L. J., M.D., L.L.B.: Doctor and Patient and the Law, Second Edition, 1949.

BIBLIOGRAPHY

Alexander; S., *et al.*: Death Following Electro-Therapy. *J.A.M.A.,* 161:0577, 1956.

Bailey, H.: Impending Death Under Anesthesia. *Brit. J. Chest Dis.,* 14:42, 1917.

Barber, R. F.; Madden, J. L.; Historical Aspects of Cardiac Resuscitation. *Am. J. Surg.,* 70:135, 1945.

Barber, R. F.; Madden, J. L.: Resuscitation of the Human Heart. *Am. J. Surg.,* 64:151, 1944.

Beck, C. S., *et al.*: Fatal Heart attack. Successful Defibrillation. *J.A.M.A.,* 161:434, 1956.

Beck, C. S.; Mautz, F. R.: Control of Heart Beat by Surgeon. *Ann. Surg.* 106:525, 1937.

Beck, C. S.; Rand, J. H.: Cardiac Arrest During Anesthesia and Surgery. *J.A.M.A.,* 141:1230, 1949.

Beck, C. S.: Resuscitation for Cardiac Standstill and Ventricular Fibrillation During Operation. *Am. J. Surg.,* 54:273, 1936.

Brofman, B., *et al.*: Electric Instability of the Heart. *Circulation,* 13:161, 1956.

Bohn, G. L.: Artificial Restoration of Cardiac Rhythm. *Brit. M. J.,* 2:725, 1939.

Bost, T. C.: Cardiac Arrest During Anesthesia. *Am. J. Surg.,* 83:135, 1952.

Cannon, W.: Voodo Death. *Am. Orthopologist,* 44:169,

1942.

Cole, F.: Use of Human Serum Albumin in Cerebral Edema Following Cardiac Arrest. *J.A.M.A.*, 147:1563, 1951.

Cole, S., and Cordey, E.: Four Minute Limit for Cardiac Resuscitation. *J.A.M.A.*, 161:1454, 1956.

Comroe, J. H.: Botelho, S.: The Unreliability of Cyanosis in the Recognition of Arterial Anoxemia. *Am. J. M. Sc.* 214:1, 1947.

Crile, G. W.: Dolley, D. H.: Experimental Research into the Resuscitation of Dogs. *J. Exper. Med.*, 8:713, 1906.

Crile, G. W.: An Autobiography. Vol. I, p. 155.

Dripps, R. D.; Kirby, C.; Johnson, J.; Erb, W. E.: Cardiac Resuscitation. *Ann. Surg.*, 127:592, 1948.

Fauteux, M.: Cardiac Resuscitation. *J. Thoracic Surg.*, 16:623, 1947.

Fink, B. R., Diffusion Anoxia. *Anesthioiology*, 16:511, 1955.

Govier, W., Vitamins in the Therapy of Shock and Anoxia. *J.A.M.A.*, 126:749, 1944.

Flagg, Paluel, The Art of Resuscitation. *Reinhold Publ. Co.* 1944.

Gurdjian, E. S.; Stone, W. E.; Webster, J. E.: Cerebral Metabolism in Hypoxia. *Arch. Neurol. & Psychiat.*, 51:422, 1944.

Harris, A. S.: Terminal Electrocardiogram Patterns. *Am. Heart. J.*, 42:895, 1948.

Harvey, W., Levine, S.: Paroxysmal Tachycardia Due to Emotion. *J.A.M.A.*, 150:479, 1950.

Hill, L.: Albutt System of Medicine. Vol. 8, p. 262, 1899.

Himwich, W. A.; *et al*: Brain Metabolism in Man. *Am.*

J. Psychiat., 103:689, 1947.

Hingson, R. A., Portable Resuscitator. *J.A.M.A.,156*:604, 1954.

Hooker, D. R.; Kowenhoven, W. B.; Langworthy, O. R.: Effect of Alternating Currents on the Heart. *Am. J. Physiol.*, 13:444, 1933.

Hosler, R. M.; Williams, J. E.: A Study of Cardioperi-cardial Adhesions. *J. Thoracic Surg.*, 5:629, 1936.

Hosler, R. M.: Cardiac Arrest from Otolaryngologist's Viewpoint. *A.M.A. Arch. Oto.*, 57:371, 1953.

Hosler, R. M.: The Emergency Treatment of Cardiac Arrest in the Operating Room. *J. Am. Nurse Anesth.*, 20:18, 1952.

Jacoby, J., *et al.*, Transtracheal Resuscitation. *J.A.M.A.*, 162:625, 1956.

Johnson, J., Kirby, C.: Cardiac Arrest. *Am. J. Surg.*, 89:56, 1955.

Johnson, J.; Kirby, C. K.: An Experimental Study of Cardiac Massage. *A. Clin. North American,* 29:1745, 1949.

Kety, S. S. *et al.*: Effects of Altered Arterial Tensions of Carbon Dioxide and Oxygen on Cerebral Blood Flow. *J. Clin. Investigation,* 27:500, 1948.

Kevorkian, J.: Fundus Oculi, Determination of Death. *Am. J. Path.*, 32:253, 1956.

Lahey, F. H.; Ruzicka, E. R.: Experiences with Cardiac Arrest. Surg. *Gynee. & Obstet.*, 90:108, 1950.

Mollison, W. A.: Heart Massage through Abdominal Incision. *Brit. J. Chest Dis.*, 14:42, 1917.

Mozen, H., *et al.*: Successful Defibrillation of Heart. *J.A.M.A.*, 162:111, 1956.

Negovski, V. A.: The Electrocardiogram During Death

and Revival. *Am. Rev. Sov. Med.*, 2:491, 1945.

Prevost, J. L.; Battelli, F.: Effects of Electrical Shock on the Hearts of Mammals. *Compt. rend. Acad. D. Sc.*, 129:1267, 1899.

Scheinburg, P.; Jayne, H. W.: Factors Influencing Cerebral Blood Flow and Metabolism. *Circulation*, 5:225, 1952.

Seldon, T. H.: Postanesthetic Encephalopathy: The Postulation of Cerebral Edema as a Basis for Rational Treatment. *Staff Meet, Mayo Clinic*, 24:370, 1949.

Shaw, C. C.: Death by Drowning. *Am. Pract. & Digest of Treatment*, 7:776, 1956.

Shenkin, H. A. *et al.*: The Effects of Change of Position Upon the Cerebral Circulation of Man. *Am. J. M. Sc.*, 216:714, 1949.

Suber, H., *et al.*: The Therapy of Carbon Dioxide Narcosis. *Am. Rev. Tuberc and Pulm Dis.*, 74:309, 1956.

Starling, E. H.; Lane, W. A.: *Lancet*, 2:1397, 1902.

Swann, H. G.: Drowning. *Tex. Rep. Biol. & Med.*, 5:423, 1947.

Wiggers, C. J.: The Interpretation and Treatment of Heart Failure During Anesthesia and Operations. *Ohio State M. J.*, 45:1169, 1949.

Wiggers, C. J.: Circulation in Health and Disease. Fifth Edition.

Wolfe, K.; Rand, J. H.: Electro-mechanical Aids in Resuscitation and Anesthesia. *Ohio State M. J.*, 46:39, 1950.

Zoll, P., *et al.*: Termination of Ventricular Fibrillation. *New England J. Med.*, 254:771, 1956.

INDEX

A

Acetylcholine, 55, 56
Acute pulmonary edema, 149
Adrenal cortex extracts, 146, 147, 149
Adrenalin (epinephrine), 37, 63, 112, 119, 124, 126, 130, 148
Age factor, 16, 48, 62
Alcohol and anesthesia, 75
Aminophyllin, 149
Anemia, 45, 51, 61, 62
Anesthesia, 78, 79
Anesthetic agents, 68, 69
Anesthetic cerebral hypoxia, 48
Anesthetist's kit, 94
Anoxia, 44, 52
Anxiety, 62
Animal experiments and demonstrations, 46, 169
Aortic compression, 127
Aristole, 163
Artificial respiration, 9, 86
Asphyxia, 8, 156, 163, 164
Aspiration of vomitus, 21, 75
Asystole (cardiac standstill)
  development, 36
  treatment, 119
Atropine, 77, 96, 141

role in hypotension without blood loss, 77

B

Bailey, H. (Hamilton), 9, 38, 199
Barber, R. F., 15, 17, 199
Basic problems in resuscitation, 17, 21, 44
Battelli, F., 10, 15, 202
Beck, C. S., 3, 11, 13, 14
Beck dictum, 101
Beck operation, 24
Blalock, A., 29
Blood
  compression bandages to prevent pooling, 146
  electrolytes, 57, 62
  pressure
    during massage, 131
    recorded, 145
    in ventricular fibrillation, 40
Body temperatures, 47, 64, 83
Boiler factory, 75
Brain damage, 147, 148
  results, 152, 153
  time limitation, 19, 46

Bronchial aspiration, 149
Bronchus, obstruction of, 150

C

Caffeine citrate, 149
Calcium chloride, 149
Carbon dioxide 71, 72, 185, 188, 191
  antianoxia action, 49
  retention, 69, 72
Cardiac arrest, 16-20
  anesthesia, 16, 26
  causes, 52-73, 169
  development of, 36-42
  types met, 30
  history of, 7-14
  incidence and statistics, 26-32
  indication of, 88, 93, 110, 111
  problems in, 17
  pulse rate, 92
Cardiac disease, 22, 58
Cardiac filling, 54, 60
  intraabdominal pressure, 61
  related to position, 59-61
Cardiac massage
  approach, 132-134
  continuation of operation, 144, 176
  history, 8, 9
  methods of, 131-140
  puncture of myocardium, 177, 178
  rate of massage, 139
  suction cup massage, 139
Case histories, 173-179
Cerebral edema, 146, 147, 153
  acute, 146

treatment, 147
Chest, closure of, 141, 144
Chloroform, 7
Chlorpromazine, 57
Circulation with massage, 131-140
Citrated blood, 57
Cleveland Heart Society Course, 14, 168
Cocaine, 13
Cole and Corday, 28
Consultation, 18, 117, 148
Continuation of operation, 144, 176
Convulsions, 69, 152
Coronary occlusion experiments, 12
Cortisone, 47, 57
Course in Resuscitation, 168
Crile, G. W., 9, 10
Cyanosis, 90
  detection of, 82

D

Death factor, 21
Death from coronary insufficiency, 23, 24, 157
Death signs, 110
Defibrillator, 97-99
  Beck-Rand type, 98
  external, 100, 101
  fire code, 99
Definition of death, 21
Dehydration, 147
Dental anesthesia, 28, 30
Drinker respirator, 145
Dripps, R. D., 200

Drowning, 160
Drugs, 54-58, 78, 79, 149
  for resuscitation, 96
  post-operative management, 149
  over-dosage, 55
Dyspnea, 150

E

Edison Institute statistics, 159
Elective cardiac arrest, 57
Electrocardiograph, 100, 148, 149
  record after death, 113
Electrocutions (accidental), 159
Electrolytic state, 62
Electromanometer, 131
Emergency act (the crisis), 101, 109, 112, 129
Emergency cart, 104
Emergency kit, 95
Errors in judgment, 63

F

Failures, 108, 121, 126, 153
Fauteux, M., 200
Fibrillation
  auricular, 38
  ventricular, 39-42
First aid, 155
Foote, M. N., 118
Francois-Franck, 13
Fundoscopic changes, 83, 110

G

Goldblatt clamp, 12

H

Heart
  beat
    observed after restoration, 141
    restoration in cardiac asystole 119, 120, 130
    restoration in ventricular fibrillation 121-126, 130
    restoration use of epinephrine, 119, 126, 130
  effect of cold, 37
  electrical stimulus, 13, 149
  manipulation of, 12, 67
  massage, 131-140
    history of, 8-10
  nerve elements, 35, 36
  stimulants (history), 10
Heart Society (Cleveland), 171
Hexamethonium, 149
Hingson, Robert, 169, 180
Holmes, Oliver Wendell, 68
Hosler, Robert, 11, 14, 168, 201
Human serum albumin, 146, 147
Hydrothorax, 150
Hypotension. 145, 146, 149
Hypothermia, 37, 47, 148
Hypoxia, 66, 90

I

Inadequate oxygenation, 89, 90
Incision, 134
Individual variation, 134
Induction, speed of, 63
Intercostal paralysis, 91
Internal mammary artery, 142

Intratracheal tube, 84, 94
  extubation, 145
Intravenous barbiturates, 68, 69
  control of convulsions, 147
Intravenous fluids, 143
Ischemic heart, 24, 42

J

Jackson, T. S., 10
Jacoby, J., 201
Johnson, J., 201

K

Kevorkian, J., 110, 201
Kowenhoven, W. B., 11, 101

L

Lahey, F. H., 201
Lane, W. A., 9, 202
Legal aspects, 195-197
  malpractice suit, 196
Levarterenol, 145
Levo-nor-epinephrine (levophed), 149
Local anesthesia, 70
Lower nephron syndrome, 148

M

Madden, J. L., 17, 199
Massage, methods, 131
Mautz, F. R., xii, 13, 199
McNamara, C. W., 173
Mechanical respirator, 103
Monitoring, 83
Morton, W., 68
Mouth to mouth breathing, 86
Mozen, H., 201

Myocardial convulsion, 39, 122
Myocardial failure, 149
Myocardium, 23, 24
  puncture of, 177

N

Necessary drugs, 96
Negovski, V. A., 201
Neosynephrine, 149
Nitrous oxide, 73
Nutritional state, 48, 62

O

Operation
  after heart beat restores, 142
  duration, 65
  type, 16
Origin of heart beat, 34
Oxygen
  and brain, 44-51
  and death, 21, 22, 44, 156
  bodily requirements, 47, 48
  extraction from blood, 50
  "system," 53
    re-establishment, 53, 107, 112-118
    breakdown of, 52
  tent, 147

P

Pacemaker, 101, 112, 149, 162
Paroxysmal tachycardia, 35, 38
Patient
  position of, 60, 80
    post-operative, 147, 150
Pericardium
  adhesions, 11, 12

closure of, 141
fenestra, 142
herniations, 142
massage with intact pericardium, 132
Picks disease (cardiac compression), 13, 142
Plasma, 141
Pneumothorax, 150
Position of patient, 60, 80
Post-operative atelectasis, 150
Post-operative management, 145-151
hematoma, 150
position, 147, 150
removal of secretions, 79, 150
temperature, 83, 148
Premedication, 57, 76, 79
Preventive measures, 74-87
coordinated action, 81
drugs, 76, 77
"fire drills," 74
instruments, 74
intubation, 84
preparation, 74, 79
Procaine, 13, 69, 76
overdosage, 69, 70, 76
Pulmonary edema, 149, 150
Pulse rate, 91, 92, 139
recorded, 145

Q
Quinidine, 149

R
Racial factors, 64
Rand-Wolfe respirator, 105

Rawolfia, 57
Reflex stimulation, 54, 66
Respiratory obstruction, 71, 91
Respiratory rate, recorded, 145
Respiratory resuscitation, 180
Respiratory stimulant, 149
Results, 152, 153
Resuscitation
cart, 104, 158
components, 5, 6
equipment for, 94-106
kit, 94
procedures, 107, 129, 130
program of action, 129
reasons for failure, 107, 108, 120
re-establishment of oxygen system, 112-118
requirements and responsibility, 3-5
restoration of heart beat, 119-130
surgical procedure, 114-118
Retinal changes, 110
Rhythm, disorders, 148

S
Safe current values, 102
Scopalamine, 77
Secret to success, 127
Seldon, T. H., 147, 202
Selman, M. W., 176
Shock, 63, 92, 143
Sinus slowing, 149
Sloan, H., 178
Starling, E. H., 9, 202
Static electricity during surgery, 28

Stephenson, H., 39
Stokes-Adams syndrome, 49, 102, 162
Subdiaphragmatic approach, 9, 132
Suction cup electrodes, 97, 126, 140
  massage, 140

T

Tachycardia, 35, 38, 42
Temperature, 83, 148
Temporary death, 13, 22
"Things Not To Do," 111
Time limit, 19, 46
Tracheal aspiration, 79, 150
Tracheal obstruction, 71, 91
Tracheostomy, 87
Transdiaphragmatic approach, 134
Transfusion
  after chest is closed, 146
  after heart beat restored, 143
  arterial, 112, 126
Transthoracic approach, 134
Trendelenberg position, 50, 59, 149

V

Vagal inhibition, 54, 148
Vago-vagal reflex, 54, 55
Variables in oxygen utilization, 46, 48
Vaso-pressor drugs, 142, 149
Ventricular fibrillation, 13, 39, 43, 158
  color of coronary arteries, 40
  condition of, 23, 40
  electric counter shock, 122
  use of epinephrine, 124
  use of procaine, 124
Ventricular premature beats, 35, 149
Ventricular tachycardia, 42, 149
Vital capacity, 58, 59

W

Whitacre, R. J., 88
Wiggers, C. J., 11, 15, 44, 202
Wolfe, K., 105, 202
Wound infections, 150

Z

Zoll, P., 101